THE
BACKYARD HERBAL
APOTHECARY

EFFECTIVE MEDICINAL REMEDIES
USING COMMONLY FOUND HERBS & PLANTS

Devon Young
FOUNDER OF NITTY GRITTY LIFE

PAGE STREET
PUBLISHING CO.

PAGE STREET
PUBLISHING CO.

First published in 2019 by
Page Street Publishing Co.
27 Congress Street, Suite 105
Salem, MA 01970
www.pagestreetpublishing.com

Distributed by Macmillan, sales in Canada by The Canadian Manda Group.

23 22 21   4 5 6

ISBN-13: 978-1-62414-746-3
ISBN-10: 1-62414-746-1

Library of Congress Control Number: 2018957772

Cover and book design by Laura Gallant for Page Street Publishing Co.

Photography by Devon Young, with contributions from Mandy Allen (pages 38, 50, 51, cover), Ann Accetta-Scott (pages 10, 72, 86, 152, 158, 159), Susan Vinskofski (pages 17, 44, 105, 166), Janet Garman (pages 104, 105, 178), Jan Berry (pages 3 and 164), Amber Reddinger (pages 11, 31, 58, 94), Ruthie Hayes (page 136), Ellen Zachos (page 82), Chris Dalziel (page 148), Quinn Veon (page 146), Colleen Codekas (page 83), and Shutterstock

Cover images © Devon Young
Printed and bound in the United States

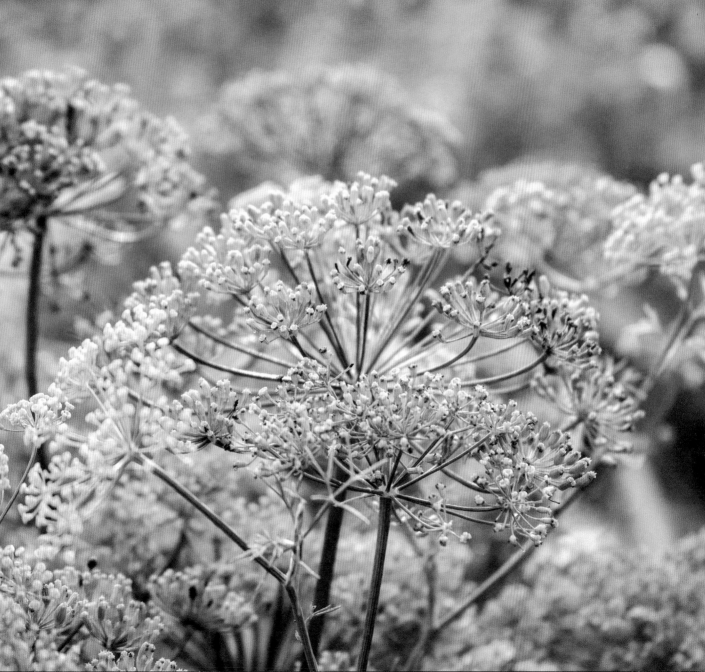

This book is dedicated to all the medicine people, wise women, herbalists, botanists and conservationists without which modern herbalism could not exist. We do not know your names or faces, but your contributions are innumerable. Your wisdom, culture and tradition should be celebrated and held in the highest regard.

 I AM HUMBLED AND FOREVER YOUR STUDENT.

CONTENTS

INTRODUCTION

Let me first tell all the budding herbalists and novice foragers that I did not grow up being taught about medicinal herbs and wild plants. There were no guided walks through the forest with a wise relative, no familial knowledge of medicinal plants to be shared with me. I was just a kid with a somewhat unusual interest in plants, raised in a family of avid gardeners. I sowed seeds and transplanted alongside my parents and grandparents every spring and summer, found joy in the harvest and browsed every issue of *Better Homes and Gardens* that came in the mail. I loved plants. I read descriptions on every nursery tag and tuned into public television gardening shows. I made daisy chain crowns and necklaces of cleavers, and I munched on the sweet blossoms of clover.

In my high school years, I considered going to school for botany, but those were the days before there was much of a push for girls in science, and my crippling lack of confidence quickly dismissed the notion. I started learning little bits here and there about medicinal herbs by checking books out from the library. I wondered if working with medicinal herbs was actually a "thing" since I only heard about naturopathy and homeopathy as some dangerous "fringe" science at the time. These were also the days before the almighty Google, so with no exposure to an herbal-ly minded holistic community, I moved on. I grew up and had kids. I experimented with herbal remedies sold at the local health food store that always smelled deliciously of curry. I worked for a couple of cosmetic companies that focused on using botanicals, and I eventually had a career in the wine industry.

I also spent these early years of my young adulthood dodging a life-threatening health crisis that the doctors could not explain, diagnose or treat. Sometimes I would just go into anaphylactic shock (conveniently, usually in the middle of the night), and these episodes seemed to have little rhyme or reason as to their cause.

After a lot of self-study and research, it eventually came to my attention that I was likely suffering from a rather extreme and frightening case of adrenal fatigue. In a nutshell, my body was allergic to stress. That saying "stress will kill you" was ringing loud and clear. Later, certain laboratory tests would indicate that my adrenal hormones, histamine levels and other contributing factors were very, very off kilter. So, what was I to do? There wasn't a proper medical diagnosis to define my condition, and the standard medical treatment (steroidal medications) of my episodes came with terrible side effects.

This is when I turned to herbal medicine and started to rebuild my health. I settled on nettle to regulate my out-of-control allergenic responses. You can see the exact tincture that I still use on page 129. I reached for yarrow to normalize my menstrual battles. Cleavers soon cleared my mess of a lymphatic system. To be clear, it was hardly an easy path to wellness. There were bumps and missteps along the way. But I found that for every troubling complaint I had, there was an herb to guide me back to health.

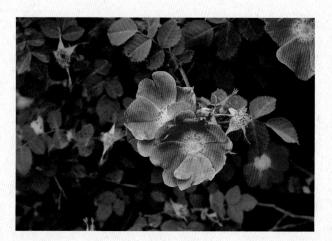

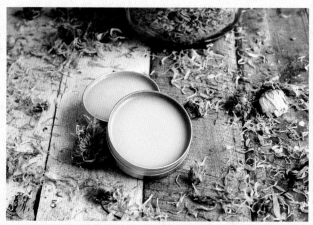

But learning herbs for myself wasn't enough. My personality being what it is, I didn't dabble. I jumped headfirst right into the deep end. I went to one of the few accredited colleges that offers a recognized degree in herbal medicine. Although my education was thorough and introduced me to the wide world of pre-clinical and clinical herbal research being conducted, I felt like there were a few elements missing. Elements like herbal energetics, folk history and usage and botanical identification.

Without these key elements, it was like looking at one small spot on an impressionist painting. Sure, it was "good stuff," but it didn't tell me all I needed to know. Borrowing concepts of herbal energetics, placing value of historical and folk usage and grasping botanical concepts helped me to stand back and see the whole proverbial "Monet."

Herbal medicine is about more than just "this herb is good for this complaint or organ." Herbs offer a broad range of medicinal use, and they invite us to engage more with our minds and bodies and, very much so, with the earth.

In this book, I want to scratch the surface on a few herbs. I want you to take the knowledge that you gain from these pages, and then experience it for yourself in the natural world. I want you to feel comfortable in knowing that you have identified the right herb and that you are using it to support your health in a profound way. I want you to make remedies with confidence and understanding. I want you to engage with the wild and cultivated landscape like you never have before.

Our plant allies don't limit their healing abilities to those with the "magic" and "instinct" to use them. If you have not received the gift of ancestral knowledge, it does not mean that you cannot have a meaningful relationship with the plant world. This book is meant to introduce you to herbal medicine, to be a gateway to the botanically-based healing in your own backyard. Each herbal profile contains traditional and evidence-based knowledge, as well as my own reflections regarding the therapeutic value of the herb so that you too can become the chief herbalist in your backyard "farmacy." You will learn about medicinal uses, how to use herbs safely, where to find them and how to grow them. I will offer you simple, effective remedies for the home apothecary that will keep you well stocked and prepared for many life events, from bee stings to ear aches, from childbirth to the loss of a loved one.

My hope is that after reading this book, you can step out into nature and see it with the curiosity of a child, the practicality of a botanist and the heart of somebody that honors the earth and its abundance.

Welcome to *The Backyard Herbal Apothecary.*

HOW TO USE THIS BOOK

As you meander down the herbal path in this book and elsewhere, you are sure to come across unfamiliar terms, concepts and practices. Do not be intimidated. This new vocabulary will soon become second nature.

The chapters of this book are titled by the most common name for the plants we are most familiar with. This may change some from locality to locality. You will also find its Latin name at the beginning of each herbal profile. It is important, especially when it comes to matters of identification and medicinal use, that we are talking about the same plant. Many plants share common names. No plants share Latin names. Make it a habit to ALWAYS confirm the Latin name of a botanical when learning a new plant. This will help you to always have your identification and use knowledge tied to the correct subject matter.

Each herb profile will also include its herbal energetics. In Western Herbalism, we suggest that people and plants have core constitutional tendencies. Some people are warm/dry, some warm/damp, while others may be cold/damp or cold/dry. You already know this about yourself, although you may not realize it. Do you sleep with the cover up around your chin? You're probably cold. Or are you the first to turn on the air conditioner when summer hits? You might be warm. Does your skin tend to feel tight after getting out of the shower? You could be dry. Or do you have clammy hands and a tendency to perspire? Maybe you are damp. Beyond our core constitution we also have tissue states. We have all felt a hot, inflamed throat, or been burdened with a mucus-y chest from a prolonged respiratory infection. Our botanical allies have these tendencies too. By selecting herbs that have the opposite actions from our constitutions or tissue states, we can take steps to returning our bodies— and even minds—to a neutral, healthy position.

As for therapeutic actions . . . this is some of the most intimidating language that you will ever encounter. *Galacto-*what? And yes, it's *alterative*, not alternative. Chances are you are about to run across some words that you don't encounter in everyday life. And for that reason, in the back of the book you can find a handy-dandy glossary of the therapeutic action terms used to give you a better snapshot of each herb's possible uses (see page 183).

Each herb will very likely have a multitude of medicinal uses, some of which may not even be mentioned in this book. In different cultures and medicinal traditions, herbs can be used in interesting, diverse ways. I have sought to present a well-rounded overview of traditional Western uses from each herb. Remember, this book is meant to provide foundational knowledge. I encourage you to learn about herbs from the many wonderful authors and folk herbalists in the world. No one person is the authority on each and every herb, and we have a practically unlimited world of plants to explore. Never stop learning! Additionally, I have included herbal substitutes for each herb. For a variety of reasons, such as accessibility or an allergy, you may not be able to use certain medicinal herbs, but that doesn't mean you simply must go without. Nature's pharmacy offers us many botanicals to choose from!

I have intentionally chosen to include simple, easy-to-follow remedies with few ingredients. I do this because the best plant medicine is that plant medicine that you *have*. As a beginner herbalist, I balked at complex formulations and techniques. How could I possibly get it right? About midway through my formal education, I found myself creating really complicated recipes. Perhaps to show off my skills and knowledge. Now a little older, a little wiser and a lot more secure in myself, I have circled back to simple remedies.

To put in bluntly: Simple is safe. Simple is effective. And simple is wise. When we use preparations with few ingredients, we know immediately what is working or not. We can make adjustments. We aren't married to the time or money that we have spent on preparing the recipe. Simple plant medicines give us freedom in our choices. Because why spend hours making a complex ointment with 50 ingredients when a simple poultice would do just as nicely? Being an herbalist should be about using the plants that are available to you in a safe and effective manner.

Please note that all the information contained in this book is for informational purposes only, and it has not been evaluated by the Food and Drug Administration (FDA). Information herein does not constitute medical advice. Please consult your physician about your particular health situation. Information presented in this book is not intended for the diagnosis, treatment or cure of any condition.

GARDENING, SUBURBAN FORAGING & WILDCRAFTING

Perhaps one of the most compelling things about becoming an herbalist is the thought of independence and the ability to take an active role in your healthcare and that of your friends and loved ones. There is something deeply satisfying about understanding how you can use the natural world to build health and wellness. The concept of purchasing my entire apothecary from manufacturers never sat well with me (although I am ever so grateful for them when it comes to herbs that I cannot grow or forage). I like to see things through from start to finish. I like to do things in a *meaningful* way. I like to grasp the whole scope of what I am doing. Perhaps you are like me. It is simply not enough for you to do the finish work. You want to learn. You yearn to create. In this modern era, some would call what we do with plants "primitive skills." I call it practical skills. Each new skill, each acquired remedy moves us closer to holistic, sustainable living.

Growing and gathering medicinal plants can be incredibly life affirming. With every seed that you sow and every leaf that you snip, you will feel more grounded and connected to nature. But I want to make emphatically clear that this is practical knowledge. Some folks speak of plants speaking to them, plants guiding them—and that is a lovely notion, most certainly. But, I would rather suggest that one must know the language of the plant kingdom before they "get" the messages plants are sending. Herbalism is learned. Plants are learned. And, unlike foreign languages, these lessons can be learned at any age, though plant language and terminology might feel a little foreign to begin with.

There are three different ways that you can stock your herbal apothecary outside of investing a great sum of money into bulk herbs and ready-made herbal preparations. Growing your herbs in your yard, foraging in neighborhoods and gathering wild medicinal plants help us to see nature through completely different eyes. No longer are we walking past a shrub, picking a flower or tugging a weed. When we learn how to identify and use herbs, we start viewing the world through a medicinal lens. And this view of the natural world is incredibly empowering. We no longer view cottonwoods as a nuisance tree that snows a cottony dander at the end of spring. Wild roses aren't just a pretty, if unkept, hedge at the edges of fields. Even the dandelion sheds its reputation as a reviled lawn pest. We no longer see these botanicals as landscape menaces and random growing things; rather, they each become a powerful plant ally with a medicinal story to tell.

GROWING MEDICINAL HERBS

It is quite likely that you are growing something in your yard or on your patio right now that has medicinal properties. Medicinal plants are everywhere once your eye is trained to see them. Even classic, well-loved culinary herbs such as rosemary and thyme have great therapeutic value. Your apothecary can literally be in your own backyard.

Growing your own medicinal herbs starts with assessing what is already in your own yard or the pots on your patio. Evergreens: Harvest the new spring tips for a rich source of vitamin C and chest-clearing qualities. Lavender: Dry some sprigs for infusing into relaxing massage oils. Do you have a vegetable garden? Try plucking corn silks for a soothing remedy for urinary tract complaints. Once your eyes are wide open to the medicinal plant world, you will start interacting with your home landscape in a totally different way.

When choosing which herbs to plant in your home landscape, you should choose herbs that are well suited to their location. Here are some considerations:

🌸 Is this herb appropriate for your climate? Will it require being moved seasonally?

🌸 Is this herb an annual, biennial or perennial for your zone?

🌸 Do you have the proper light conditions (full sun, part shade, full shade) for this herb?

🌸 Do you have the best soil conditions (dry and arid, heavy clay, sandy loam, deep and rich) for this herb?

🌸 Can you provide adequate water for this plant?

🌸 Is this herb considered a noxious weed in your area?

🌸 Will this herb be aggressive or prone to problems in your yard?

🌸 Do you have adequate space for this plant?

🌸 Is the planting of this herb prohibited by any community associations or governing bodies?

A well-thought-out home landscape can offer a variety of attractive and medicinal plants. Growing your own herbal medicine also allows you to know the conditions that the plants were exposed to throughout the growth cycle, such as pesticide and herbicide application on or near the plant, soil contamination risk, possible animal contamination and other qualitative concerns. Additionally, the mere proximity to the plant helps to ensure that you never miss the ideal harvesting window. Although your yard may be limited in some capacity, there is a medicinal herb for practically every size and type of landscape!

FORAGING THE NEIGHBORHOOD AND URBAN AREAS

Stepping out of your own yard and exploring your surrounding neighborhood can be a truly enlightening experience. Discovering useful botanicals in your surrounding area is one of the most sustainable and ecologically sound ways of practicing herbalism! Does your neighbor have sunny calendula spilling out of a garden bed? Are there spires of mullein at the edges of the park? Are petite little daisies dotting the elementary school lawn? There is often more abundance in these traditionally cultivated landscapes than first meets the eye. A side benefit of foraging your neighborhood and urban areas is the conversations and introductions these actions create. Ask an elderly neighbor if you can dig the dandelions in her side yard, and you surely have a friend for life. Inquire with a nearby school about picking up their black walnuts as they drop. You are sure to draw the affections of the custodians and groundskeepers. Even abandoned homesites often yield an incredible biodiversity of interesting and medicinal plants.

Of course, it is not a free-for-all. There are some very important factors to weigh, such as:

🌸 Do you have express permission to gather and harvest from the property owner?

🌸 Did you offer compensation in some way for use of somebody else's yard? I usually offer to share some of the remedy I am making.

🌸 Can you take adequate measures to ensure that you minimize impact to another person's property?

Is this area free from pesticide and herbicide residue? How has this plant been tended in this yard? While it is not necessary for the plants to be cared for to the letter of organic farming practices, chemical fertilizers, pesticides and herbicides use should be avoided on or near the plant.

Could the site have contaminated groundwater or soil? This is often the case with industrial sites; do not harvest.

Are these plants free from pet waste?

Is the plant at least 50 feet (15 m) from a major roadway?

What is the source of your plant? Fresh from the nursery stock is often loaded with chemical fertilizers, as well as having an increased risk of pesticide and herbicide contamination. I wait at least a year before harvesting from nursery stock for medicinal purposes.

By taking a few precautions into account and having conversations with you neighbors and property owners/managers, you will go a long way to fostering great relations in your community. While some people might raise an eyebrow as you gather up clingy cleavers, just as many will be glad to see their plants have a new use and will take interest in what you are doing.

GATHERING WILD MEDICINALS

Though I generally try to shy away from overly romantic notions, gathering herbs in their wild habitat nourishes my soul in ways that I cannot adequately explain in words. And I know that I am far from alone in this feeling. There is something very meditative and calming about engaging with nature and removing ourselves from the trappings of modern society. The sounds of insects, birds, breezes and rushing waters replace the sounds of mobile device notifications, televisions and vehicles. The rhythm of identifying, inspecting and collecting each herb takes the place of racing thoughts and monkey-brained machinations. Is that a violet tucked under that fern? Can I get to that mugwort on the other stream bank without getting too wet? Can I harvest just enough elderflower now so that there will still be plenty of berries come fall?

Wildcrafting takes a trained eye to notice the subtleties in leaf and flower. It also takes some careful forethought, preparation and planning to do correctly and respectfully.

Such considerations are:

Are you harvesting a plant that is considered threatened or at risk?

Can you harvest this plant and still leave enough of this plant in the surrounding area for it to continue to thrive? It is not recommended to harvest over 30 percent of any "stand" of an herb, with many conservationists recommending no more than 10 percent.

Are you properly equipped and clothed to deal with terrain and weather conditions?

Can your harvest be processed in a timely manner?

Can you correctly spot at least three major identification markers for each plant you are gathering?

Do you have knowledge of harmful and toxic look-alikes?

Can you preserve a small portion of this plant material for reference in case of emergency due to false identification so that medical personnel can determine the proper mode of treatment?

Is it legal for you to harvest this plant or from this land?

Wildcrafting can be very rewarding when performed with knowledge and respect. Novice wildcrafters may find helpful allies in seasoned hunters, as they are often familiar with the boundaries of public lands and private lands that you can obtain permission to harvest from, and they may even have a strong working knowledge of plants in your area. Local farmers are also a good resource, especially when it comes to identifying plants that an herbalist may find useful but are toxic to grazing livestock.

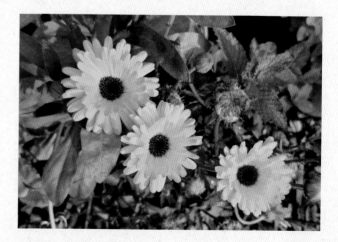

KEY IDENTIFICATION TERMS

While the notion of the "language of plants" may sound quite romantic and conjure images of plants swaying softly in the breeze while a woman in a gauzy tunic kneels close by, I would argue that the language of plants is far more pragmatic. In fact, there is a language very specific to *how* we describe plants. Botanical terms give us a common language to share.

Why is it important to share a common plant language, you ask?

Well, it is the same reason that we always reference the Latin name when speaking scientifically about plants. Different words, names and terms mean different things to different people. That can create confusion when speaking to somebody from another locality or culture or when using a different language. Using key botany terms to describe plants leads to more accurate descriptions, which leads to more accurate identifications. Accurate identifications make for safe and effective remedies. After all, that is what we are seeking: safe, effective remedies from clearly identified, trusted plant allies.

Here is a primer on some of the botany terms that you will see used in this book to describe leaves, flowers, stems and other plant parts used in the "Identify & Grow" keys for each herb:

ALTERNATE LEAVES: leaves arranged in an alternate pattern along the stem (see raspberry leaves, page 172)

BASAL LEAVES: leaves arise from a clump (see first year mullein, page 64)

OPPOSITE LEAVES: leaves arranged directly across from each other on the stem (see chickweed, page 82)

WHORLED LEAVES (AND FLOWERS): leaves or flowers radiate around the stem (see self heal flowers, page 42)

RACEME: spike-like flower cluster (see black cohosh, page 136)

UMBEL: flower clusters with stems radiating from a central stem, usually roughly equal in length, create a flat to slightly rounded flower head (see elder, page 16)

PINNATE: feather-like; leaflets arranged on either side of stem, often opposite (see black walnut, page 104)

PALMATE: maple leaf–like; lobes of leaves arranged on both sides of a midrib (see hawthorn, page 88 and Oregon grape, page 38)

SIMPLE: leaf is not heavily dissected; even if somewhat lobed, the leaf is not cut to the midrib (see comfrey, page 30)

COMPOUND: several distinct leaf parts joined at a central stem (see black cohosh, page 136)

BI-, TRI-, ETC. FOLIATE: denotes number of leaves

BI-, TRI-, ETC. PINNATE: denotes number of divisions in leaves with pinnate arrangement

SERRATED, TOOTHED: margins of the leaf have a jagged edge (see wild rose, page 120)

DISSECTED, DIVIDED: lobes of the leaf are deeply cut (see black cohosh, page 136)

STIPULES: leaf-like protrusions at the base of a leaf stem

BRACTS: a modified leaf

PISTIL: female reproductive organ of the flower

STAMEN: male reproductive organ of the flower

PETALS: individual segments of the flower "corolla"; often colorful

SEPALS: leaf-like parts that enclose the flower bud

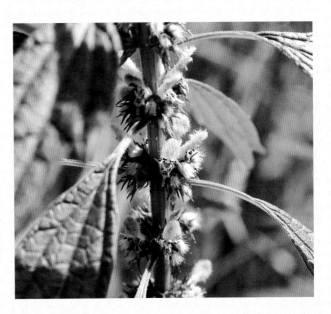

HERBAL PREPARATIONS

Consensus among herbalists is a moving target. We are an independent bunch. One can find that herbal preparation terms differ somewhat from herbalist to herbalist. For the purposes of this book and my blog, the following terms are reflective of their following definition.

TEA: A tea is prepared with dried herbs that are steeped in hot water for 5 to 10 minutes, then strained and consumed. They are typically prepared from leaves and flowers. Teas are best for minor acute complaints, and they have a pleasing flavor.

HOT INFUSION: Hot infusions are prepared like teas, but stronger and for longer. Typically steeping for a minimum of 20 minutes before serving, hot infusions have a bolder flavor and more prominent tannic and bitter notes. Hot infusions that are allowed to steep and cool for at least 12 hours are considered "nourishing herbal infusions (aka Sunsun Weed)." Infusions tend to have more nutritive and medicinal value. Roots and dried berries, as well as mineral-rich leaves, such as nettle, benefit from the prolonged extraction time. Hot infusions that have been cooled are also great for applying as a compress.

COLD INFUSION: Cold infusions are ideal for extracting mucilage—a thick, viscous substance that has the ability to coat—found in herbs such as marshmallow. Cold infusions are prepared by steeping dried herbs in cool water for 6 to 12 hours before straining and serving.

OIL INFUSION: Herbally infused oils are great as massage oils and as the bases of other creations. There are several ways to infuse oils, typically with dried or well-wilted herbs unless otherwise specified:

REGULAR INFUSION: Herbs are infused in a chosen base oil for a minimum of 6 to 8 weeks (typically in a cool, relatively dark place) before being strained and bottled or prepared into further remedies. This is a preferred method for well-dried herbs, especially for those with delicate aromatics that could be destroyed by heat. This is an excellent method, although it does take a substantial amount of time.

SOLAR INFUSION: Oils are prepared as with the regular method but taken to a bright sunny location, such as a south-facing windowsill, to infuse during the day. The increase in heat helps to extract stubborn constituents, but some feel as though the base oil suffers degradation due to ultraviolet light exposure. There also is increased probability for accidents and breakage in the frequent handling, as it is not advisable to leave solar infusions outdoors overnight because a drop of temperature may promote condensation and potentiate spoilage.

HEATED INFUSION: In this method, herbs and oils are prepared as one would for the solar or regular infusion, but the jar is placed in a water bath in a slow cooker at its lowest setting for 24 to 72 hours typically. This method is fast and excellent at extracting more resinous constituents. This is not ideal for herbs with more delicate aromatics.

DOUBLE BOILER METHOD: This method uses a double boiler set up to rapidly infuse an oil in about an hour or less. This is great method for fresh plant material as it allows for moisture to escape. Be sure to watch this method closely to ensure that the herbs and oil do not overheat and that the bottom pan does not boil dry.

DECOCTION: Roots and bark, as well as certain fungi, are often prepared as a decoction to fully extract constituents from woody and fibrous plant material. Herbs and oils are simmered at a low boil until the volume is reduced by half, then strained before serving.

TINCTURE: Tinctures are typically alcohol based, although some tinctures can be prepared with vinegar or vegetable glycerin. These bases are referred to as the *menstruum*. I use each menstruum for specific reasons, such as:

HIGH (190) PROOF: Spirits with a very high level of alcohol are appropriate for resinous material, such as cottonwood buds and pitch/sap.

MEDIUM (100) PROOF: I use medium-proof spirits for tincturing fresh berries and whole flowers.

LOW (80) PROOF: Lower-proof spirits are most appropriate for leaves and dried plant matter.

VINEGAR: This is an excellent menstruum for extracting minerals from herbs such as nettle and horsetail.

VEGETABLE GLYCERIN: While it is somewhat of a weak menstruum, glycerin is ideal for those who object to or abstain from alcohol. It is also useful for children because its sweet taste increases compliance. This preparation is best suited for more delicate plant material such as leaves and flowers.

OXYMEL: An oxymel is a vinegar- and honey-based preparation for internal use. Oxymels are a great way to prepare berries and other highly aromatic/flavorful herbs.

SYRUP: Often prepared from leaves, flowers and berries, herbal syrups are based on either a simple or "thick" syrup recipe. Simple syrups are made in a 1:1 sugar to water ratio, while thick syrups are made in a 2:1 sugar to water ratio. Thick syrups are relatively stable at room temperature, while simple syrups should be refrigerated.

POULTICE: A poultice is a mash of fresh herbs, or dried herbs with water, applied, to an infected area and wrapped with a cloth. Poultices are typically prepared from leaves.

PLASTER: Similar to a poultice, dried ground herbs, usually leaves and flowers, are mixed with flour and warm water, then worked into a paste and applied to a cloth and set on an affected area, often with a hot water bottle placed on top to increase the therapeutic benefits.

SUCCUS: A succus is a preparation in which fresh leaves and/or flowers have been juiced or blended with a small amount of water or another aqueous substance such as aloe.

SALVE/BALM: These are semi-solid preparations in which an infused oil is hardened with beeswax. Salves/balms can be applied directly to areas of concern such as minor scrapes, burns and abrasions.

OINTMENT: These are similar to salves but include a tincture or extract to increase the medicinal aspect of the preparation.

SERUM: I generally refer to serums as non-oil-based preparations for external application. Serums may contain herb-infused vegetable glycerin, aloe and even seaweed gels as the base.

CREAM/LOTION: These are oil- and water-based emulsions that are held in suspension with emulsifying wax. Please note that beeswax and other waxes often produce inconsistent suspensions. Creams are thicker and more emollient, whereas lotions are thinner, often with a "pumpable" consistency. Due to the high water content of creams and lotions, they must be refrigerated or a preservative must be used to deter microbial contamination.

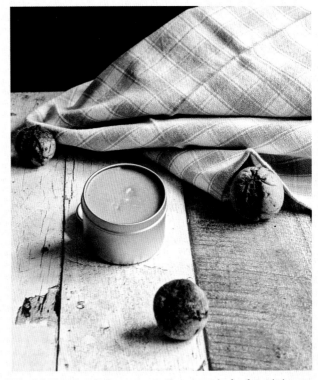

This black walnut salve is an excellent remedy for fungal skin complaints (page 106).

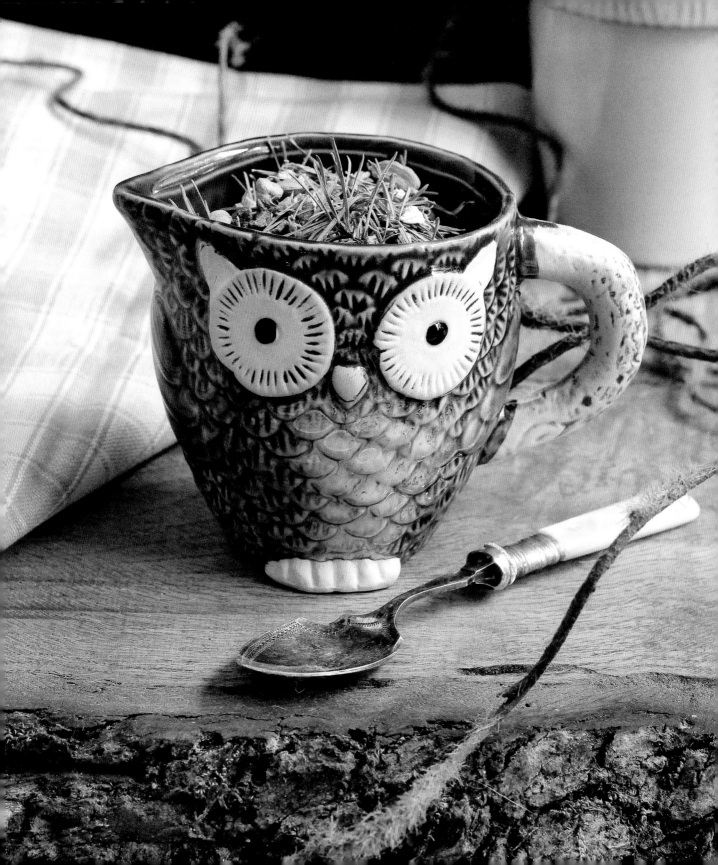

HEALING FOREST AND MEADOW DWELLERS

THE FOREST IS A MOSAIC OF MEDICINE, slowly revealing the botanical bounty hidden in the canopy, tucked away in the understory and peeking out from the shaded meadows. Follow a trail through the woods, and you'll observe a scene not unlike an impressionist painting—shades of green and earthy brown, dappled with delicate whites, pinks and purples all painted with nature's feathery brushstrokes. A calm and patient eye will soon see that this place of quiet and peace is a botanical wonderland of lichens, leaves, needles, berries, bark and roots offering gentle healing and nourishment.

Explore the woods and find medicine around every bend in the trail. Reach into the canopy and gather the citrusy lime green fir tips in spring for a fragrant respiratory ally. Keep your eyes to the ground as you enter the dappled sun of the meadow to discover sweet little self heal, known for its restorative and protective actions on the skin, hidden in the grassy areas between the trees each summer. Dig deep into the earth at the forest's edge come fall to collect the luminous yellow roots of Oregon grape, whose roots are one of nature's most profound medicines for the liver. Dust aside the winter snows to trim a few fragrant cedar boughs for the clean, clear sense that the graceful tree evokes.

Forest medicine awaits discovery.

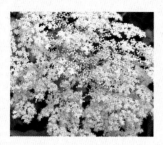

ELDER

OTHER COMMON NAMES: elderberry, elderflower

LATIN NAME: *Sambucus nigra, S. canadensis*

HERBAL ENERGETICS: cool/dry

THERAPEUTIC ACTIONS: anti-inflammatory (berries), antioxidant, antiviral, astringent (flowers), diaphoretic (flowers), diuretic (flowers), immune-modulating, nervine, refrigerant

PARTS USED: flower & berry

HERBAL MONOGRAPH

The storied elder tree has a bounty of beautiful medicine contained at the tips of its boughs. This makes it a fantastic herb for beginners, and it's why I chose this plant for the first medicine that I purposely produced years ago: an elderberry tincture, using fresh berries infused in brandy, studded with a bit of cinnamon and ginger. Sadly, the berries were slightly underripe and the tincture barely palatable. You live, you learn. I have since honed my elder skills, my tincture now rivals a fine sipping liqueur and my arsenal of elder medicine has greatly increased.

Folkloric tradition abounds with elder use. It is a botanical associated with charms, superstition, spells and symbolism. Placed over a threshold, woven into a wreath and sometimes avoided altogether, elder has an air of magic and mysticism. Chiefly linked to protection, superstition sheds much light on elder medicine.

The first elder virtues to arrive are in the form of the flower. Frothy white umbels of tiny star-shaped flowers arrive during the final weeks of spring in northern climates. These delicately fragrant blossoms behold a wealth of medicine. Elderflowers are unmistakably cooling, energetically speaking and they are best applied to hot, overstimulated conditions. A principal use of elderflower is that of a fever reliever. Elderflower is specifically suited to those fevers in which the individual is hot and agitated, radiating heat. It is not the appropriate choice for the individual that has a fever accompanied by chills. A hot, sour stomach and digestive tract often will also benefit from the cooling nature of this herb.

For all its apparent delicacy, elderflower is a robust antiviral herb. Considering both its heat-clearing and antiviral attributes, elderflower is the foremost herb that I reach for when there are complaints of the flu with fever and irritability. It is also called for with other viral complaints such as Epstein-Barr, mononucleosis, chicken pox and shingles. Not only does elderflower address the heat and viral components of the illness, its nervine qualities soothe the overarching sense of agitation and neediness. It is, without a doubt, my favorite herb for dealing with small children: compresses of an elderflower infusion can even be applied to a fussy, teething infant to soothe and calm the child.

As the seasons progress, the almighty elder delivers its second crop of medicine in the waning days of summer and early fall. Those delicate umbels of white foam-like blossoms give way to small berries in shades of blue and black, which have come to be known as one of the most renowned immune supporting botanicals in the herbal medicine world. Elderberry taken throughout the typical "cold and flu season" is a widely accepted preventative protocol, although the evidence of its efficacy is somewhat anecdotal. Elderberry remedies taken at the onset of flu symptoms have drawn quite a bit of scientific attention with several studies indicating that they help to drastically reduce both the duration and severity of symptoms such as fever, cough, running nose and body ache. Traditional herbalists point to the use of elderberry for croupy coughs, coughs that become worse at night and deep lung congestion.

The value of elderberries is not limited to viral issues and complaints of the lungs. Due to its high anthocyanin content, elderberries support cardiovascular health in a variety of ways. A study of 21 healthy volunteers in 2014 examined the blood lipid profiles of each individual after consuming 200 milliliters of elderberry infusion over a course of 30 days. The results indicated scientifically significant reductions in triglycerides, low density lipoproteins (LDL) and overall cholesterol levels.

BEST PREPARATIONS: The flowers and berries of the elder tree lend themselves to a variety of medicinal and culinary recipes. The flowers can be tinctured either fresh or dried in alcohol or glycerin—the latter being particularly child friendly. Dried flowers make lovely teas and infusions, alone or in concert with other herbs. The flowers make a delightful syrup that can be drizzled over cakes and used to sweeten cocktails and mocktails alike. Other culinary applications for the flowers include fritters and candies.

Ripe elderberries can also be tinctured fresh or dried. The berries also make the most delicious syrup that can be prepared on its own or with other immune system supporting herbs. I particularly like using elderberries in an oxymel preparation: a vinegar and honey mixture that not only tastes good but

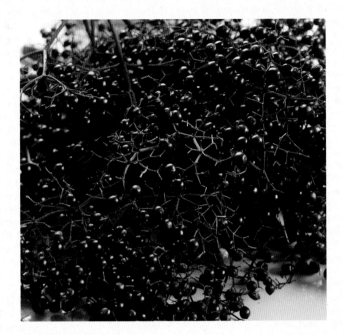

IDENTIFY & GROW

❀ **TYPE OF PLANT:** Deciduous tree or shrub

❀ **HABITAT:** Elders are found in a variety of places, but they are most at home in an open wooded setting with sandy loam soils that do not become extremely parched even during extended periods of no rain.

❀ **HEIGHT:** Typically 4–12' (1–4 m)

❀ **LEAF:** 5 to 7 finely toothed lance-shaped leaves, pinnately arranged. Most often the foliage is green, although domesticated cultivars now appear with dark burgundy foliage.

❀ **STEM:** Hollow

❀ **FLOWER:** Large umbels of small white flowers approximately 4–12" (10–30 cm) across appearing late spring to early summer

❀ **FRUIT:** Blue (with a white bloom or haze) to purple-black depending on species; ripens in late summer through early fall

❀ **GROWING INFORMATION:** There are a variety of cultivars that lend themselves particularly well to the home landscape, including a few that are quite showy and beautiful. Elders should be planted in a semi-protected area not prone to high winds, as their brittle stems can snap in heavy gusts. Take care to water your elder frequently during establishment, and water your larger specimens during drought. Do not prune newly planted elders until well established. Some cultivars will require two different species of elder for pollination.

❀ **FORAGE OR GROW?** With all the beautiful cultivars available, this is a great medicinal botanical to grow. Elders can be found throughout most temperate regions and are not difficult to identify, making this an easy herb to forage.

BEST HARVEST PRACTICES

FLOWER HARVEST WINDOW: Late spring to early summer

BERRY HARVEST WINDOW: Late summer to early fall

When harvesting flowers, keep in mind that by snipping the blossom head you are reducing the fall berry crop. Harvest the flowers modestly. Take care only to harvest ripe berries. Note: The stems of both the flowers and berries may cause digestive upset and should be carefully removed before using.

triggers a strong salivary response which promotes the appetite. Elderberry candies, such as lollipops, are a clever way to deliver the herb's benefits to a reluctant child. The berries make lovely wines, cordials, jams and chutneys.

HERBAL SUBSTITUTES: Astragalus (*Astragalus membranaceus*): immune support | hawthorn berry (*Crataegus* spp.): cardiovascular | catmint (*Nepeta cataria*): diaphoretic

SAFETY AND PRECAUTIONS

Both elderflowers and berries are widely regarded as safe. However, if you are pregnant or nursing, or taking prescription medication, you should consult your physician before using this or any other herb.

There is some concern about the use of elderberries for those suffering with autoimmune issues. There seems to be little cohesive scientific or anecdotal evidence to strongly support or negate their use in these persons. I personally take this to mean that some autoimmune sufferers may experience flare-ups while others may not, and that it is largely individual to each person. If you do have an autoimmune disorder, please consult your specialist before using this or any other immune supporting or modulating herb.

Although some older sources indicate some medicinal value, the leaves and bark of elder trees are considered toxic. Avoid unripe berries, as they contain a cyanic glycoside until they are fully mature. Some sources also suggest heating the berries before use to ensure no toxic traces remain.

ELDERFLOWER GLYCERITE FOR FEVERISH WEE ONES

My experience as a parent is that fevers always spike at bedtime. My kids will always doddle about with a low-grade fever during the day, only to get super toasty at night. My youngest likes to produce fevers that would bust the top right off an old-school thermometer. I generally see a fever as a powerful part of the immune process that should not be suppressed. Low-grade fevers are an important part of the immune response and help the body's natural defense. However, it is important to discuss with your physician when a fever is entering some potentially scary territory. For those fevers that are uncomfortably high, leaving little ones in a perpetually fussy state and parents on edge, this elderflower glycerite gently cools the heat and promotes much needed rest for all.

Elderflowers are naturally cooling with a delicate, sweet, floral flavor. Vegetable glycerin is naturally sweet and viscous, which helps to ensure compliance when administering the glycerite.

YIELD: 4 ounces (about 120 ml)

CHILD'S DOSE, AGES 2–6: 1–2 droppers (1.5–3 ml), every 3 to 4 hours as needed

CHILD'S DOSE, AGES 6–12: 1–2 teaspoons (5–10 ml), every 3 to 4 hours as needed

INGREDIENTS

4 oz (120 ml) organic vegetable glycerin

¼ cup (5 g) fresh elderflower blossoms (flowers removed from stems)

INSTRUCTIONS

Add the vegetable glycerin and elderflowers to a small jar with a tight-fitting lid. Infuse the glycerin with the elderflower for a minimum of 6 weeks. After the infusion is complete, strain through a fine-mesh sieve into a liquid measuring cup. Pour into 1- or 2-ounce (30- or 60-ml) amber glass dropper bottles. Use within 1 year.

NOTE: An alcohol-based elderflower tincture may be more effective for teens and adults. You can make this by infusing 1½ cups (30 g) elderflowers in 2 cups (480 ml) 100 proof spirits for approximately 6 weeks. Strain and bottle. Adult/teen dose: 1–3 droppers full (1.5–4.5 ml)

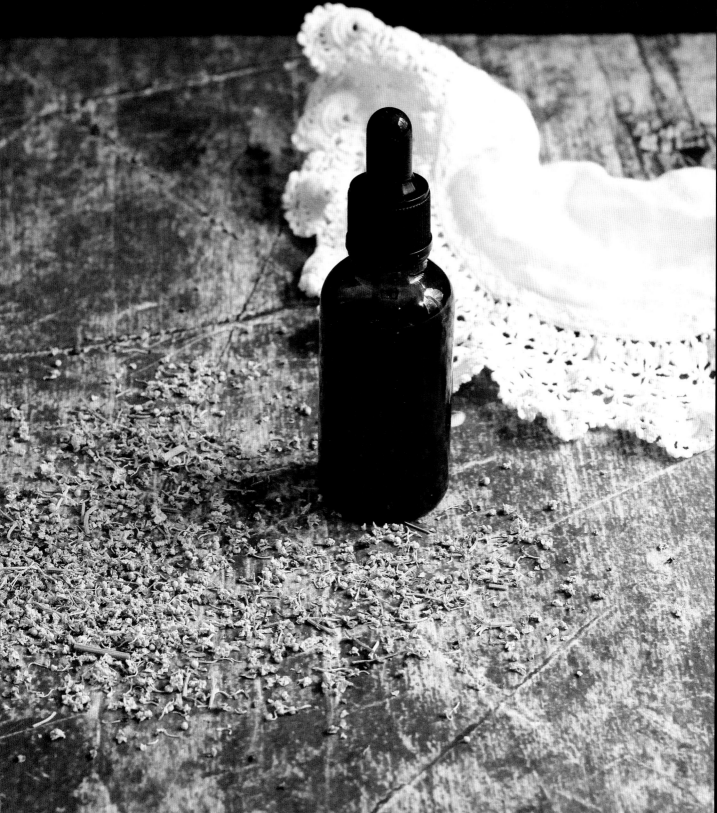

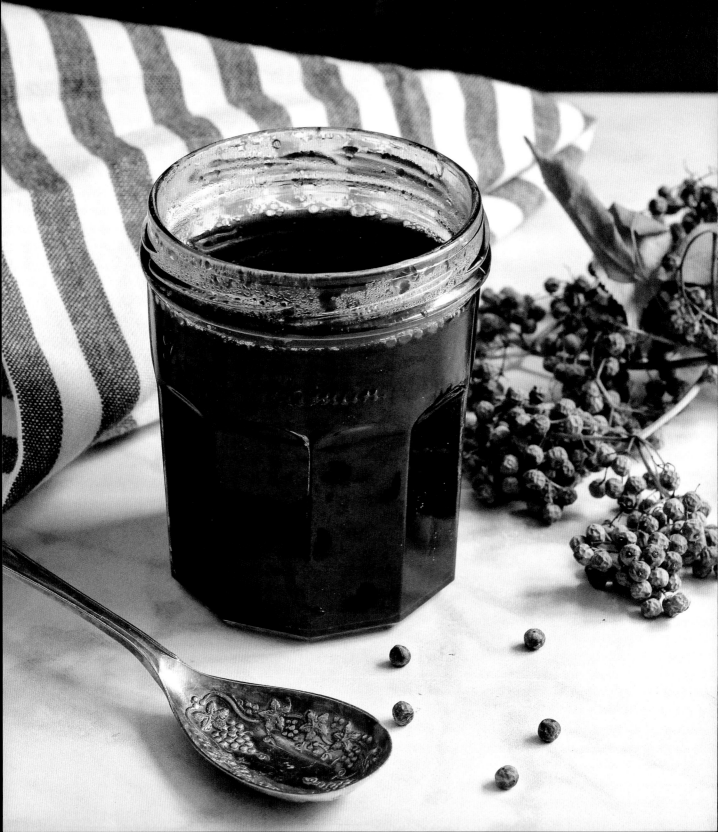

TANGY & SWEET ELDERBERRY OXYMEL FOR IMMUNITY SUPPORT

Oxymel sounds kind of esoteric and potion-y, right? Coming from the Latin words for *acid* and *honey*, an oxymel is really just vinegar and honey. This becomes a highly medicinal blend when we add herbs such as elderberries. And in the case of elderberries, this blend becomes rather tasty too!

This elderberry oxymel is crafted with raw apple cider vinegar and unfiltered raw honey to increase the health benefits of this flavorful concoction. This oxymel can be administered as a medicinal syrup or added to sparkling water or cocktails as a refreshing beverage and is a tangy and sweet way to support the immune system on a daily basis.

YIELD: approximately 1 quart (1 L)

ADULT DOSE: 1–2 tablespoons (15–30 ml), 3–4 times daily

CHILD'S DOSE, AGES 2–12: ½–2 teaspoons (2.5–10 ml), 2–4 times daily

INGREDIENTS

2 cups (480 ml) raw apple cider vinegar

1 cup (145 g) ripe fresh elderberries

2 cups (480 ml) raw, unfiltered honey

INSTRUCTIONS

Combine the vinegar and elderberries in a jar with a tight-fitting lid. If using a metal lid, use a slip of parchment paper between the lid and the jar to prevent rust from forming. Infuse the vinegar with the elderberries for a minimum of 2 weeks. After the infusion is complete, strain through a fine-mesh sieve into a small bowl or large liquid measuring cup. Add the honey to the infused vinegar, and stir well to combine. Pour into a quart-sized (1-L) bottle and store in the refrigerator. Use within 1 month.

> **TIP:** If the ripeness of your fresh berries is somewhat questionable, or if you are concerned about elderberry safety, gently heat the vinegar/berry infusion to a simmer. Cool completely before straining and combining with honey.

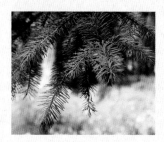

FIR

OTHER COMMON NAMES: grand fir, noble fir, balsam fir (all *Abies* species)

LATIN NAME: *Abies* sp.

HERBAL ENERGETICS: cool/dry

THERAPEUTIC ACTIONS: anti-inflammatory, antimicrobial, antioxidant, anti-rheumatic, antiseptic, antispasmodic, diuretic, expectorant, hepatic, sedative, vulnerary

PARTS USED: needles

HERBAL MONOGRAPH

Fir trees are steeped in Native American folklore and tradition. Fir trees are closely associated with protection across many Native cultures. Northwestern tribes, particularly the Salish, used fir for cleansing and spiritual matters. Other North American tribes used firs for weather magic and sleep. Pitch, needles and bark were all part of Native American medicinal practices and tradition.

Firs are known for their aromatic qualities. A hike through an evergreen forest often leaves one feeling restored and invigorated. This sense of rejuvenation is owed to its aromatics. The volatile compounds of the fir needles promote deep, fully actualized breaths and a subtle sedative (think more meditative than sleepy) quality. This "forest therapy" extends beyond the woods and into the apothecary. Fir needles, consumed as a tea or infusion or even applied as an infused oil, speed relief to tight, swollen airways, heavy boggy chests and irritable coughs.

Fir needles have long been used by Native Americans and early settlers to address rheumatic and gout complaints. As a diuretic, it helps to flush excessive fluids built up in the tissues, resulting in relief to swollen and painful joints. Similarly, fir needles help to moderate water retention and puffiness. Fir needles also have an affinity for the liver, offering protective, antioxidant actions.

Fir sap or pitch has been used for impromptu bandages for minor cuts, but is even more effective for irritations. When the sticky resin is applied to bug bites, it helps to calm the redness and itch. Similarly, when gently dabbed on a sliver or an embedded stinger, covered with a small cloth or leaf, and then gently removed, it will often lift the irritant from the skin and provide immediate relief!

BEST PREPARATIONS: Fir needles offer an intriguing balsamic and citrusy note to teas and infusions. Fir-infused oils make a lovely base for massage oils, salves and lotion-making.

Spring fir tips have a delightfully citrusy flavor and texture, making them suitable for food. I have even made a forest-y pesto with fresh needles that I slather on freshly caught trout before grilling. Fall needles are a bit sturdier and require a fine chop, but they impart a rich balsamic note to baked goods and syrups.

HERBAL SUBSTITUTES: Rosemary (*Rosmarinus officinalis*): respiratory | Douglas fir (*Pseudotsuga menziesii*): respiratory

SAFETY AND PRECAUTIONS

Fir needles are generally considered safe for internal and external use. If you are pregnant, nursing or taking prescription medication, please consult your physician before using this or any other herb.

LOOK-ALIKES: Douglas fir (*Pseudotsuga menziesii*)

IDENTIFY & GROW

TYPE OF PLANT: Coniferous tree

HABITAT: Fir trees are typically native to mid- and high elevations, although they are often found near sea level. Firs prefer well-drained soils, and they will not survive in boggy conditions.

HEIGHT: 30–250' (10–80 m)

LEAF: Very slim needles, somewhat soft and flat in shades of green to silvery blue

STEM: Twigs have a smooth bark

FRUIT: Cones that are ovoid with flexible scales

GROWING INFORMATION: Plant firs in well-drained soil with plenty of room to expand in both height and width.

FORAGE OR GROW? Firs are easily identified in their native habitat, while also making beautiful, long-lived trees for the landscape. One can easily forage from wild trees or gather from a neighborhood giant.

BEST HARVEST PRACTICES

FIR TIP HARVEST WINDOW: Spring to early summer, depending on climate and elevation

Needles can be gathered at any time, but the spring growth is more tender and brighter in flavor. Needles harvested later will be tougher and more balsamic in flavor (which is still quite nice). Do not harvest from small or diseased trees.

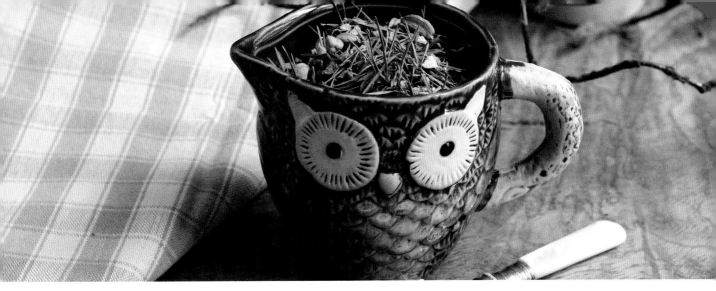

FOREST-TEA CHAI FOR RESPIRATORY WELLNESS

I really love the flavor of fir tips—citrusy, balsamic and resinous without being bitter. Combined with some traditional chai spices, this blend smells and tastes like the holidays. But more than that stellar flavor and aromatic wonder, the fir tips, orange and spices open the chest and sinuses to help one breathe deeply. I find this tea to be most comforting when my chest feels heavy and my stomach unsettled, with sinuses that feel painful with applied pressure.

Gather fir tips in the spring and dry thoroughly to ensure you have an adequate, shelf-stable supply of the needles for this tea and other preparations.

YIELD: approximately 3 cups (280 g) of dried tea blend

INGREDIENTS

2 cups (100 g) dried fir tips

2 tbsp (15 g) dried orange zest

2 tbsp (15 g) cinnamon chips

2 tbsp (15 g) green cardamom pods, lightly crushed

2 tbsp (15 g) star anise pods, lightly crushed

2 tbsp (15 g) dried ginger granules, lightly crushed

1 tsp black peppercorn, lightly crushed

Raw honey, to taste (optional)

INSTRUCTIONS

Combine the fir tips, orange zest, cinnamon chips, cardamom pods, star anise pods, ginger and peppercorn and store in a jar with a tight-fitting lid in a cool, dark place. Use within 1 year.

Prepare the tea by steeping 1 heaping tablespoon (5 to 7 g) of the mixture in 8 to 10 ounces (240 to 300 ml) of water just off the boil. Infuse for 5 to 7 minutes or longer if desired, then strain into a serving mug. Sweeten with raw honey, if desired.

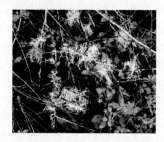

USNEA

OTHER COMMON NAMES: old man's beard, lungs of the forest, beard moss, bread lichen

LATIN NAME: *Usnea* sp.

HERBAL ENERGETICS: cool/dry

THERAPEUTIC ACTIONS: analgesic, antibacterial, antifungal, anti-inflammatory, antiparasitic, astringent, styptic, tonic, vulnerary

PARTS USED: whole plant

HERBAL MONOGRAPH

Among the limbs of the canopy above, usnea can often be found in small nest-like tufts or long elegant strands. Usnea is an herbal medicine that has earned a permanent place in my home apothecary. For many complaints, I find that usnea delivers when conventional, modern practices fail.

With a common name like "lungs of the forest" it should not come as a surprise that usnea is an herb with respiratory applications. As an aerial botanical, usnea thrives only in areas of pristine clean air. It has an ability to clear our airways of wet, heavy congestion and hot, painful conditions. Usnea is a unique antimicrobial agent with an ability to inhibit the cellular metabolism of both gram-positive and gram-negative bacteria. As such, usnea may benefit those suffering with an infection of the respiratory system caused by bacteria such as *Mycobacterium tuberculosis*, *Pseudomonas aeruginosa*, *Staphylococcus* and *Streptococcus*.

Usnea is also particularly effective for complaints of the urinary and digestive tracts. When there are concerns of candida overgrowth, usnic acid—an active constituent of usnea—has demonstrated the clear ability to alter the morphology and encourage cell death in a strain of *Candida albicans*. Furthermore, usnic acid is effective against *Bacillus cereus* and most strains of *Escherichia coli*, making usnea a possible remedy to foodborne illnesses and some urinary tract infections. Some sources also indicate that usnea may be an effective remedy for protozoan parasitic infection of *Trichomonas*.

Because usnea is a profound infection fighter, as well as anti-inflammatory styptic agent, this lichen is considered forest first aid for wounds and insect bites. Used as a poultice or packed onto fresh wounds, usnea has great potential in moments of crisis when conventional care may be elusive.

BEST PREPARATIONS: Usnea is most effective when tinctured. While some herbalists suggest a high-proof alcohol extraction using 190 proof spirits, I tend to prefer slower extractions using 100 proof spirits over a longer length of time (six months to a year). Usnea can be infused into a base oil to create medicinal ointments, and it can be dried and powdered for spot wound treatment.

HERBAL SUBSTITUTES: Bee propolis: antimicrobial | Oregon grape (*Mahonia aquifolium*): antimicrobial

SAFETY AND PRECAUTIONS

Usnea is generally regarded as safe by the herbal community, even for younger children and the elderly. If you are pregnant, nursing or taking prescription medication, please consult your physician before using this herb. It should be noted that high concentrations of usnic acid may cause liver damage, but these concentrations cannot be achieved in the home using the whole herb and standard tincturing methods.

LOOK-ALIKES: There are many varieties of lichen that can be confused, such as Spanish moss (*Tillandsia usneoides*). Identify usnea by the white, stretchy, inner filament.

IDENTIFY & GROW

🌼 **TYPE OF PLANT:** Lichen

🌼 **HABITAT:** Usnea is often found on the bark and limbs of coniferous trees, although it can be also found on deciduous trees throughout the world. Depending on the species, it can grow small palm-size tufts or long strands.

🌼 **STEM:** Usnea has a gray-green stem-like structure. If you pull away the outer coating, you will reveal a white, elastic filament which is characteristic to this lichen.

🌼 **GROWING INFORMATION:** I know of no way to plant or propagate this lichen.

🌼 **FORAGE OR GROW?** This is an herb to forage.

BEST HARVEST PRACTICES

LICHEN HARVEST WINDOW: Fall and spring to take advantage of windfall due to storms

As some particular species are somewhat slow growing, it is best to only harvest windfall, unless usnea is otherwise abundant to the area. Usnea should only be foraged in clean, contamination-free areas as it is a bio-accumulator of lead and other heavy metals, as well as environmental pollutants.

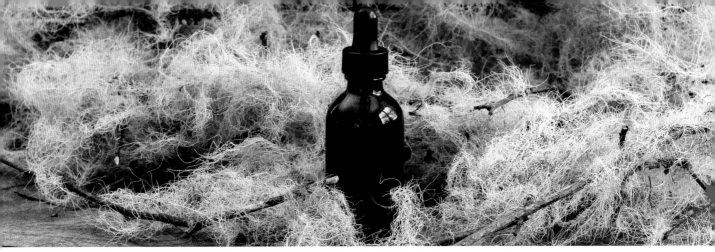

USNEA DUAL EXTRACTION TINCTURE FOR RESPIRATORY COMPLAINTS

Let's get one thing clear: lichens are kind of weird. With one foot in the plant world and another in the fungus world, lichens require a bit of patience and effort to take advantage of all their medicinal virtues. This preparation requires two types of extraction—one in alcohol and another in water. Then these two extracts are married and preserved with vegetable glycerin, making an excellent tincture for respiratory complaints.

I tend to think of usnea as my herbal antibiotic, and I use this when there are complaints indicative of respiratory and urinary infections and inflammation. I often use adjunct therapies, such as aromatics (like the Forest-Tea Chai for Respiratory Wellness, page 23) and demulcents (like marshmallow or corn silk), to increase comfort and well-being while usnea does the infection-fighting dirty work.

YIELD: approximately 1 pint (480 ml)

ADULT DOSE: 1–3 droppers full (1.5–4.5 ml), 3 times daily

CHILD'S DOSE, AGES 6–12: 1 dropper full (1.5 ml), 3 times daily

CHILD'S DOSE, AGES 2–6: 15 drops, 3 times daily

INGREDIENTS

1 cup (240 ml) 100 proof spirits

½ cup (45 g) firmly packed fresh usnea

2 cups (480 ml) distilled water

2½ oz (75 ml) vegetable glycerin

INSTRUCTIONS

Combine the spirits and usnea in a jar with a tight-fitting lid. Infuse for a minimum of 6 weeks, shaking daily. After the infusion is complete, strain through two layers of flour sack cloth into a liquid measuring cup, saving the tinctured usnea. Set the filtered tincture aside.

Transfer the tinctured usnea plant matter to a small saucepan and add 2 cups (480 ml) of water. Prepare a decoction by simmering over medium heat until the liquid is reduced by half, about 20 to 30 minutes. Cool completely and strain the decoction into a liquid measuring cup.

Combine the tincture and decoction and stir in the vegetable glycerin. Stir well to combine. Pour into 1- or 2-ounce (30- or 60-ml) amber glass dropper bottles or into a pint-sized (480-ml) amber glass bottle for dispensing. Use within 1 year.

WILD GINGER

OTHER COMMON NAMES: Canadian snakeroot

LATIN NAME: *Asarum canadense, A. caudatum*

HERBAL ENERGETICS: warm/dry

THERAPEUTIC ACTIONS: alterative, anti-inflammatory, antimicrobial, antispasmodic, cardiovascular stimulant, carminative, diaphoretic, digestive, diuretic, emmenagogue, expectorant

PARTS USED: root

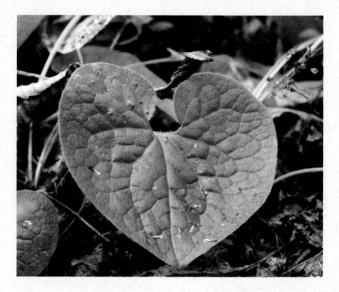

HERBAL MONOGRAPH

It seems to go without saying the use of herbal medicine often invites lively discussion and outright controversy at times. This is very true in the "us versus them" scenario that pits herbal medicine against modern, conventional medicine. I personally feel that the two modalities can be used simultaneously for a truly holistic approach to healthcare. But even within the greater herbal community, we see disagreement on any number of subjects. This is especially true with regard to wild ginger. Despite a strong ethnobotanical history of use by Native Americans, as well as early settlers and explorers, wild ginger garnered scorn in the early 1990s. Wild ginger was deemed toxic, a "do not use" herb.

Before we tread into the territory of the medicinal value of wild ginger, it is important to understand the context of its bad reputation so that you can make an informed decision about its place in your home apothecary. I would argue that the controversy surrounding wild ginger use is a case of a few bad apples spoiling the barrel with a heaping dose of equating isolated constituent use with whole herb use—they are not one and the same.

This embattled botanical first drew the ire of the medical and herbal community in early 1990s when a cousin of wild ginger, *Aristolochia fangchi*, was included as an ingredient in diet pills. I know. Hold the phone: diet pills in the 1990s were toxic. Those times were certainly a perfect storm of dangerous beauty standards, a largely unregulated "supplements" industry throughout North America and most of Europe, and unethical manufacturers motivated by greed. Sadly, 105 users of this diet supplement were stricken with acute renal failure, over half of which required kidney transplants. This and subsequent similar incidents led researchers to surmise that the constituent aristolochic acid, which is present in varying amounts in many wild ginger species including *A. canadense*, was toxic. It should be noted that *A. caudatum* contains barely traceable amounts.

Further research then confirmed that aristolochic acid indeed causes kidney damage and may contribute to increased cancer risk. While these findings are grave, there are a few factors to consider. Formal research conducted on lab animals used high doses of an isolated constituent injected directly into animal tissue—essentially bypassing the buffering effects of the digestive system. These factors are difficult, if not impossible, to replicate in the home apothecary, and they are totally outside of the scope of traditional herbalism.

The horrifying experience suffered by those who took the diet pills has very little to do with wild ginger use in practice. While the potential for toxicity with this herb is most certainly an area for concern, arguments can be made in favor of safe and well-thought-out wild ginger use, employing whole herb preparation in the proper menstruum.

Wild ginger, much like traditional culinary ginger, is very warming and stimulating. As a diaphoretic, it is ideally suited for those with fevers paired with cold, clammy skin, paleness and chills. Its spicy pungency is also welcome when there are complaints of a wet cough that is persistent and nagging. Applied in the form of a salve or paste to the chest, wild ginger helps stimulate and encourage expectoration. Taken internally as a tea, it will dry excessive mucus and ease an upset stomach due to sinus drainage.

There is a strong tradition of using wild ginger for women's health concerns. Wild ginger encourages blood flow to the pelvic area, warming and stimulating the uterus, making it quite useful for damp, boggy conditions and a sense of perpetual fullness about the lower abdomen. The botanical is used to bring on a delayed menses and soothe menstrual cramping. It also has been used in midwifery to ease a woman through the passage of a miscarriage or to re-invigorate a stalled or slowly progressing labor (often used in low doses in conjunction with black cohosh).

Wild ginger can be incredibly effective for lessening the pain associated with muscle spasms, as well as arthritic and rheumatic conditions. It warms and soothes cold, stiff joints, puffy, fluid-filled pockets and tight, clenched muscles by speeding blood flow to affected areas.

I feel strongly called to plead the case for wild ginger. This is an abundantly useful herb—one with benefits that outweigh any alleged risk when used appropriately. It also serves as an important reminder that plant medicine should be respected. You may have heard before that anything that has the potential to heal has the potential to harm. That is the case with wild ginger—but proper preparation mitigates or even eliminates these risks.

BEST PREPARATIONS: Due to toxicity concerns, extra precautions must be considered when using wild ginger. Both ethanol (alcohol) and acetic acid (vinegar) extract aristolochic acid quite readily. To mitigate aristolochic acid extraction, many herbalists would recommend preparing wild ginger as a tea or infusion. A decoction of the root can be prepared, strained and preserved with a 10 percent dilution of 195 spirits, which can then be used as a low-dose tincture (2 to 5 drops, as needed). Oil infusions for massage or for salve making are another suitable preparation for wild ginger.

Dried wild ginger root can be used as a substitute for culinary ginger, contributing a more complex, woodsier flavor.

HERBAL SUBSTITUTES: Ginger (*Zingiber offinale*): stimulant

SAFETY AND PRECAUTIONS:
Use with caution (see earlier references). Do not use if you have kidney disease. If you are pregnant, nursing or taking prescription medication, please consult with a physician before using this or another herb.

LOOK-ALIKES: Rue anemone (*Thalictrum thalictroides*) TOXIC

IDENTIFY & GROW

TYPE OF PLANT: Perennial

HABITAT: Wild ginger is a low-growing perennial that prefers dense to dappled shade in rich, moist soils.

HEIGHT: 6" (15 cm)

LEAF: Velvety, kidney bean–shaped to heart-shaped with heavy veining; leaves appear in pairs. Usually green, with some cultivars appearing variegated and slightly blue toned.

FLOWER: Flowers appear below the leaf canopy, barely above the soil surface. The flower consists of three fused sepals that are green at the base, becoming bronze-red at the tips, which can be quite spreading and divergent. Blooms appear in April and May.

ROOT: Rhizome has a distinct ginger aroma.

GROWING INFORMATION: Wild ginger is most successfully propagated by root division in early spring. This plant requires ample shade and is intolerant of drought-like conditions. This plant can be divided in the wild and transplanted to the home garden. I have also found it as nursery stock, especially at nurseries specializing in native plants. There are even variegated varieties for extra visual interest. Given the choice, I would select the safer *A. caudatum* for the medicinal garden.

FORAGE OR GROW? Although it would take a keen eye to spot wild ginger in the dense understory of the forest floor, this botanical often grows in creeping mats and has a very characteristic odor, making it very identifiable. It is also well suited to the shady home garden, creating an attractive ground cover. This botanical can be either foraged or grown if the right conditions exist in your yard.

BEST HARVEST PRACTICES
ROOT HARVEST WINDOW: Late summer to early fall

Lift the roots by fall, before the plant goes dormant. Roots should be cleaned, sliced and dried for future use.

WARMING WILD GINGER RUB FOR THICK & HEAVY CHESTS

This warming chest rub is sure to get stubborn chest congestion moving. The peppery, spicy aroma will clear your sinuses and bring healing circulation to a cold, clammy chest wall—all without the camphor-y burn of commercial chest rubs!

It is important to use dried wild ginger for this oil infusion to reduce the risk of spoilage due to moisture content. Fresh rhizomes can be harvested and cleaned, chopped into small pieces and laid out in a dehydrator or a warm oven until fully dried and brittle. The dried rhizome can then be used for this salve and tea making.

YIELD: 8 ounces (240 ml)

INGREDIENTS

½ cup (45 g) dried wild ginger root

1 cup (240 ml) base oil blend of your choice (I like coconut oil and olive oil)

2–4 tbsp (20–40 g) beeswax pastilles

INSTRUCTIONS

Using the regular or heated oil infusion method (page 12), infuse the wild ginger into the base oils. After the oil is adequately infused, strain through muslin or cheese cloth.

Return the oil to a double boiler, add the beeswax, then warm until completely melted. Remove the oil-beeswax mixture from the heat. Pour into individual 2-ounce (60-ml) containers, approximately 4, or other similarly sized jars. Allow to cool completely before putting a lid on the container. Use within 1 year.

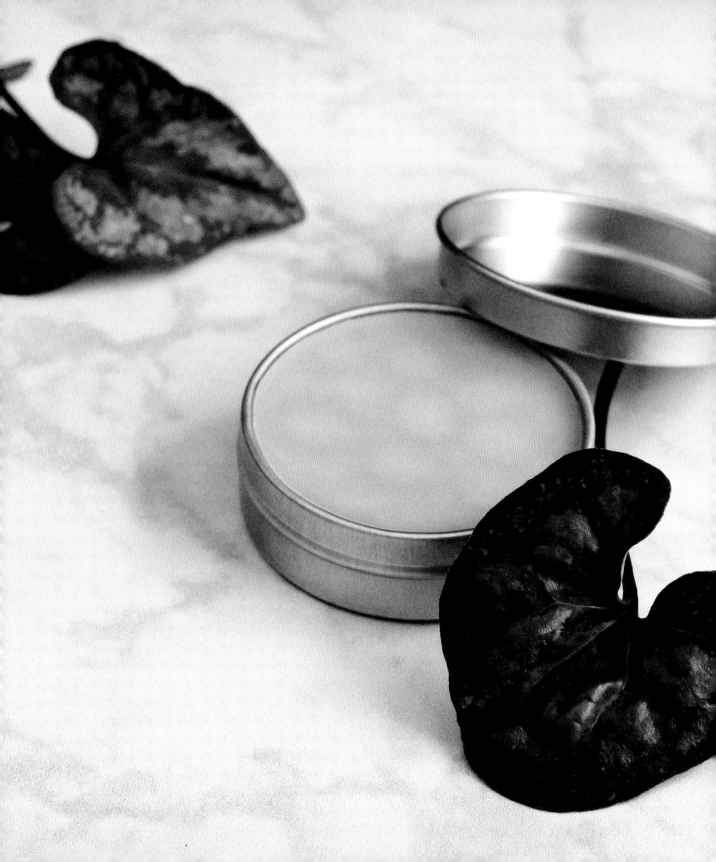

COMFREY

OTHER COMMON NAMES: knitbone, boneset, healing-herb

LATIN NAME: *Symphytum officinale*

HERBAL ENERGETICS: cool/moist

THERAPEUTIC ACTIONS: alterative, anti-inflammatory, astringent, cell proliferant, demulcent, expectorant, nutritive, styptic, tonic, vulnerary

PARTS USED: leaves, flowering tops, roots (external use only)

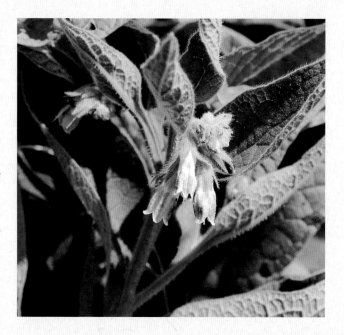

HERBAL MONOGRAPH

Comfrey is the great mender of all things broken.

From broken skin to fractured bones, this is a botanical known for its ability to stitch the torn and tattered body back together. Sometimes, when I look at a plant, its very appearance sheds light on its uses. Comfrey is characterized by large leaves—the kind of leaves that blanket, wrap and protect, but perhaps not in a way that you would expect. These leaves would not be considered soft, rather, they have a texture not unlike a cat's tongue. But maybe its rough texture sheds light on its value. Comfrey is an old medicine, and it is a workhorse, but it isn't a soft, cuddly, use-it-all-the-time medicine. Comfrey is a battle-hardened field medic.

Older botanical common names usually give us an indication of its use, and comfrey is no exception. The names knitbone and boneset (also a shared common name) suggest that comfrey has an innate ability to repair and weave together the inner cellular matrix. Ancient Greek materia medicas offer up comfrey as a healer of wounds and broken bones as early as 50 CE. Even the botanical name, *Symphytum*, derives from the prefix sympho-, meaning "to unite."

While history teaches us of comfrey's application in all matters of broken bone, considering effective modern splinting and casting, our uses for comfrey are slightly less dramatic. But comfrey remains incredibly useful, often filling the gap where conventional medicine leaves us wanting. I find comfrey to be indispensable for all manner of sports injuries, especially those of jammed and swollen fingers and toes. Comfrey seems to draw down swelling and pain while simultaneously bringing flexibility and mobility to the affected area. As such, the application of comfrey is perfect for sprained, strained, jammed or broken fingers and toes. Moreover, I find this herb to be one of the precious few herbs that can relieve the pain and expedite the healing of broken ribs.

Comfrey's ability to knit together all that is broken is not limited to bone, tendon and ligament. Few herbs match its ability to bring healing to the largest organ of our body—our skin. Comfrey encourages the growth of new cells while also providing moisture, ameliorating inflammation and softening hardened tissues. A 2012 study found that an oil/water emulsion (a lotion) containing 8 percent comfrey leaf extract to be an extremely effective wound healer in rats. In fact, comfrey is so effective at promoting wound closure by urging on the production of new skin cells, that it can be too effective for infected wounds, requiring the use of antimicrobial herbs such as yarrow and Saint John's wort to make a well-balanced salve. Comfrey salves and ointments are particularly effective for dried, chapped hands, rough skin, abrasions and minor cuts, and it may also be helpful for bedsores when no infection is present.

No discussion of comfrey would be complete without a thoughtful and frank discussion regarding its internal use. Older texts point to comfrey to address a whole variety of complaints such as cough, sore throat, stomach ulcers, heartburn and intestinal complaints. It is a known and effective soother of mucus membranes. That being said, there is some controversial evidence to suggest that internal use of comfrey may contribute to liver damage by way of one of its pyrrolizidine alkaloid (PA) constituents. It should be noted, first and foremost, that PAs are concentrated mostly in comfrey roots, with little to no PAs present in the leaves, stems or flowering tops. Additionally, some sources indicate that PAs are destroyed at high temperatures in the preparation of infusions and decoctions. Still others suggest that the study that points to the potential for toxicity was flawed in that the rat subjects were exposed to exceptionally high amounts of PAs daily for extended lengths of time, over 2 years, and that the study was not indicative of rational medicinal use and didn't account for the short life span of lab rats, typically 2 to 3 years. Those arguments aside, the herbal community is staying on the safe side of the comfrey-use debate. Current recommendations are for external use only.

BEST PREPARATIONS: Comfrey is an excellent herb to apply as a poultice, either fresh or dried. A cooled infusion is also excellent as a compress. Comfrey makes an exceptionally soothing infused oil that can be used to craft ointments and salves.

HERBAL SUBSTITUTES: Calendula (*Calendula officinalis*): wound closure | gravel root (*Eupatorium purpureum*): bone health

SAFETY AND PRECAUTIONS
Comfrey should be for external purposes only. Do not use comfrey on a wound with an active infection.

LOOK-ALIKES: Foxglove (*Digitalis* sp.) TOXIC

IDENTIFY & GROW

TYPE OF PLANT: Perennial

HABITAT: Comfrey is adaptive to a multitude of conditions. It prefers moist, rich soil, but due to its long tap roots, comfrey is fairly drought resistant. Comfrey prefers neutral pH soils and partial to full sun.

HEIGHT: 3–4' (1–1.2 m)

LEAF: Simple, alternate leaves are rough, hairy and broad with pronounced veining

STEM: Hairy

FLOWER: Pendulous, bell- or funnel-shaped flowers in shades of white, pink or purple arising on a long stem from a leaf axis. Flowers are small and five-petaled, with a tubular throat.

GROWING INFORMATION: Comfrey grows well in a variety of conditions, but will thrive in an area of moderately rich soil that has an ample supply of water without being perpetually damp. Comfrey may be difficult to grow from seed, as it requires cold stratification and has an exceptionally long potential germination ration of up to two years.

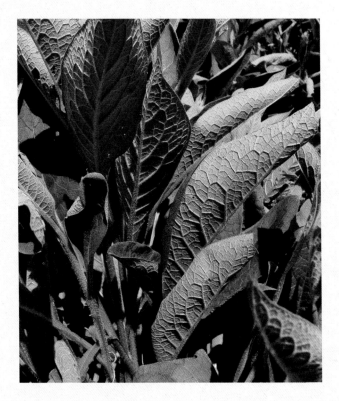

FORAGE OR GROW? As comfrey is an attractive plant and fairly disease resistant, it is an herb that is at home in the cultivated landscape. It also bears some resemblance to toxic foxglove, so make certain that your identification is 100 percent accurate.

BEST HARVEST PRACTICES
LEAF AND FLOWERING TOP HARVEST WINDOW: Summer

ROOT HARVEST WINDOW: Fall

Leaves and flowering tops can be collected and dried quickly during the growing season. I like to hang-dry the long stems in a cool, dark and low-humidity environment. In the fall, roots can be dug, cleaned, sliced and dried.

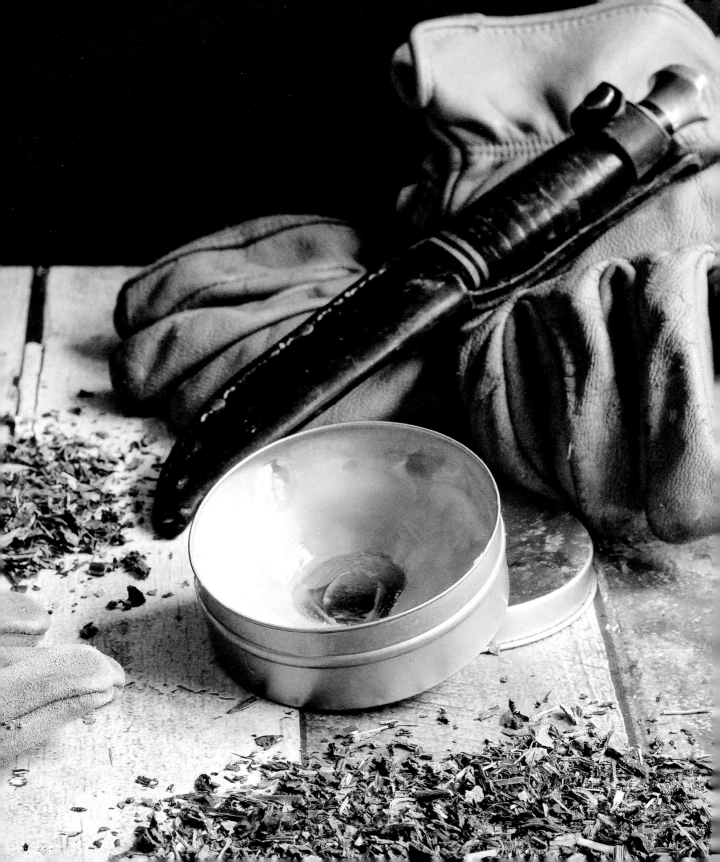

COMFREY SALVE FOR ROUGH, HARDWORKING HANDS

There are hardworking hands, and then there are HARDWORKING HANDS. The grizzled, stained, chapped and calloused paws of farmers, mechanics, masons, carpenters and other professionals and hobbyists are always in need of some tender loving care. This comfrey salve is perfect. Not only does it help to soften hardened and cracked hands, it also offers relief from inflammation and pain in tired, overworked and strained joints.

YIELD: approximately 8 ounces (240 ml)

INGREDIENTS

¼ cup (13 g) dried comfrey leaf

¼ cup (25 g) dried comfrey root

1 cup (240 ml) base oil blend of your choice (I like coconut oil and olive oil)

2–4 tbsp (20–40 g) beeswax pastilles

50 drops essential oil(s) (optional)

INSTRUCTIONS

Using the regular or heated oil infusion method (page 12), infuse the comfrey leaf and root into the base oils. After the oil is adequately infused, strain through muslin or cheese cloth.

Return the oil to a double boiler, add the beeswax and warm until completely melted. Remove the oil-beeswax mixture from the heat, and stir in essential oils, if desired. Pour into individual 2-ounce (60-ml) containers, approximately 4, or other similarly sized jars. Allow to cool completely before putting a lid on the container. Use within 1 year.

TIP: Comfrey is incredibly effective for sprains and strains when made into a poultice wrap. When one of my daughters once came home with a visibly swollen finger that had been jammed, I applied a comfrey poultice and within 30 minutes, her pain had greatly lessened and there was no longer any visible swelling. Plainly put, this is an easy remedy that works. Simply bruise a fresh comfrey leaf using an ice mallet, rolling pin or pestle. Wrap the leaf around the affected area, and secure with gauze or medicinal tape. To use dried comfrey leaves, mix the comfrey with a small amount of water, smear the paste on the area and wrap securely with gauze. For either method, let the poultice sit in direct contact with the skin for 30 to 60 minutes, and reapply if necessary.

FALSE CEDAR

OTHER COMMON NAMES: arborvitae, red cedar, white cedar

LATIN NAME: *Thuja occidentalis, T. plicata*

HERBAL ENERGETICS: warm/dry

THERAPEUTIC ACTIONS: anthelmintic, antimicrobial, antiperspirant, antiseptic, astringent, decongestant, deodorant, diuretic, emmenagogue, expectorant, lymphatic, stimulant

PARTS USED: leaf (scale-like needles)

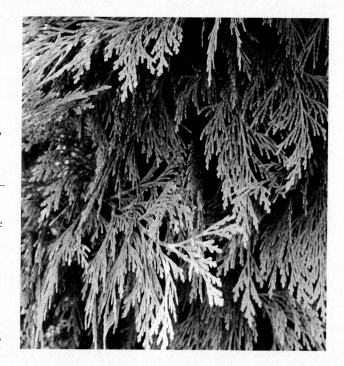

HERBAL MONOGRAPH

Known as the "Tree of Life," North American cedars are remarkable trees of stature and grand presence. While not technically "cedars" (true cedars are native to the Mediterranean), these towering giants are actually members of the cypress family, but will be referred to here as cedars for the sake of simplicity. North American cedars hold a place in ceremony, tradition and medicine in many Native cultures. The trees are often associated with purification and protection, and they are often used in sweat lodge ceremonies and medicine making. Perhaps the most iconic use of cedars is the finely detailed totem poles of the Pacific Northwest.

The medicinal value of North American cedars is as great as their presence. Cedar medicine is powerful medicine. Cedar acts on the kidneys and urinary tract in a very profound way. In what seems somewhat contradictory, cedar is considered a diuretic, but is indicated for issues of incontinence and weak bladder/pelvic floor. Cedar seems to encourage full evacuation upon urination, while also stimulating and toning the bladder muscles and pelvic area. Cedar is often suggested for those who experience bladder leakage upon exertion (including sneezing, laughing and coughing) and from enlarged prostate, as well as for children with a tendency to wet the bed. As a powerful antimicrobial agent, cedar is suggested for urinary tract infection. Note that cedar is too stimulating for those with debilitated kidneys due to disease.

Cedar has long been associated with cleanliness and purity. Its scent is a natural bug repellant, and it is often used to line closets and linen chests. Its highly aromatic qualities also make it a great consideration for soap and deodorant making. As a member of the cypress family, cedar helps to regulate sweating, making it especially helpful for those with a tendency to underarm wetness, while also mitigating the bacteria that cause body odor. Cedar serves as a popular botanical for those prone to acne with oily skin that has a waxy appearance, and homeopathic *thuja* is often suggested for those with chronic and persistent acne. Cedar has also been used to address complaints of warts, ringworm and thrush (yeast infections).

Native American cedar is an effective, stimulating expectorant for those with cold, wet conditions of the upper respiratory systems. The volatile, highly aromatic oils of this mighty tree seem to loosen and thin stubborn bound-up mucus and encourage drainage. As a lymphatic, cedar will also help to soften swollen and tender nodes about the neck.

TIP: Swags of cedar draped across mantles or along bannisters are not only beautiful holiday décor, but offer great respiratory benefits.

BEST PREPARATIONS: Due to its aromatic nature, cedar is an excellent herb for external uses such as herbal steams and oil infusion for salves, massage and soap making. Internal use should be limited to teas and infusions. Tinctures of cedar can be produced but must only be used as a low-dose preparation due to the relatively high thujone content. Cedar swags make for aromatic décor, and incense and smudge sticks can be burned for a pleasing aroma.

HERBAL SUBSTITUTES: Fir (*Abies* sp.): decongestant

SAFETY AND PRECAUTIONS
Do not use false cedar if you have kidney disease. If you are pregnant, nursing or taking prescription medication, please consult your physician before using this or any other herb.

LOOK-ALIKES: Asian *Thuja* species

IDENTIFY & GROW

🌸 **TYPE OF PLANT:** Coniferous tree

🌸 **HABITAT:** North American cedars are adaptable and grow in a variety of areas. They are often found in mixed fir and hemlock forests on hillsides and flat land, as well as mountainsides and marshland. They are even reproductive under dense shade.

🌸 **HEIGHT:** 10–200' (3–60 m)

🌸 **LEAF:** Flattened, fan-shaped branchlets with scale-like needles

🌸 **TRUNK:** Bark is somewhat fibrous and has a tendency to peel from the trunk in thread-like strands. Western red-cedar bark has a noticeable red tint.

🌸 **GROWING INFORMATION:** North American cedar tolerates various conditions and is quite hardy. Domesticated cultivars, called arborvitae, are especially fast growing and have a columnar habitat, making for excellent hedges and privacy shields in residential areas.

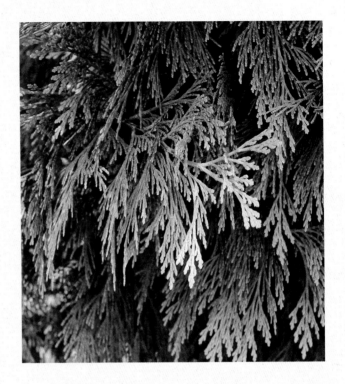

🌸 **FORAGE OR GROW?** Cedars are plentiful in nature and easily identified. They also make excellent landscape trees providing shade and privacy from neighbors in a very short time. As such, these trees are an equally great choice for both foraging and growing.

BEST HARVEST PRACTICES
HARVEST WINDOW: Cedar branchlets and needles can be collected throughout the year.

EVERGREEN CEDAR COLD PROCESS SOAP

Soapmaking was one of the big DIY projects that I was too anxious to try for the longest time. Until one day I finally did it and fell in love with the process. This cedar-infused soap is very lightly scented by the needles, but delivers great cleansing and healing action. This soap is also considered "super-fatted"—meaning that it has slightly more oil than is used up by the lye during the saponification process, making it a very gentle soap when fully cured.

When handling lye, take appropriate safety precautions. Keep children and pets out of the soap making area and wear gloves, long sleeves and safety glasses. Always keep some vinegar at the ready to neutralize any lye spills. Note that all measurements except for the essential oil are given by weight; a digital scale is needed to safely make soap from scratch. You will also need a soap mold, dedicated immersion blender and a plastic basin to catch any spills when preparing and cooling the lye solution.

YIELD: approximately 2½ pounds (1.1 kg)

INGREDIENTS

12½ oz (370 ml) olive oil

12½ oz (354 g) coconut oil

2½ oz (75 ml) castor oil

2½ oz (71 g) cocoa, mango or shea butter

Hot water

2¼ cups (90 g) fresh or dried cedar needles, divided

4.13 oz (117 g) lye granules

1–2 tbsp (15–30 ml) essential oil of your choice, optional (I like cedarwood and pine or sage)

INSTRUCTIONS

Infuse the olive oil, coconut oil, castor oil and cocoa butter with 2 cups (80 g) of cedar needles using the heated infusion method (page 12). When the infusion is complete, strain the oil through two layers of flour sack cloth and set aside in a tight-lidded jar until ready for soap making. Before soap making, reweigh the oil and adjust with more or less oils so that the oil weight is exactly 30 ounces (890 ml).

Prepare a "cedar tea" with approximately 1½ cups (360 ml) of hot water and ¼ cup (10 g) of cedar needles. Cool to room temperature (or colder in the refrigerator). Strain the tea, and measure out 10 ounces (300 ml) of the cedar tea.

Wearing safety gear (long sleeves, rubber gloves and protective eyewear), prepare your lye solution in a plastic tub with the recycle symbol #5 on it. I use this so that it can be thrown away. Carefully pour the premeasured lye granules into the cooled cedar tea. After working with your lye, wipe up the area with a paper towel dampened with vinegar to clean and neutralize any stray lye granules. Your lye solution will superheat to near boiling point and may discolor (don't worry). Place a lid on the container and cool in a safe and secure spot until the lye solution is about 90 to 110°F (32 to 43°C).

Meanwhile, warm the infused oil to 90 to 110°F (32 to 43°C). When both mixtures are approximately 90 to 110°F (32 to 43°C), transfer the oil to a heavy crock or stainless-steel bowl (do not use aluminum). Slowly pour the lye solution into the oil, using an immersion blender to emulsify. Make sure the blender stays below the mixture to avoid splatter. Within a couple of minutes the mixture will reach the "trace" stage when an instrument dragged through the mixture leaves an impression before settling in. Add the essential oil at this time, if using, and blend thoroughly.

Quickly pour into a parchment- or silicone-lined mold. Smooth the top with a rubber spatula. Wrap the mold in a couple layers of towels. Cool in a safe spot for 24 to 36 hours. Unmold and cut to the desired thickness. Note that slightly thinner soaps will cure faster. Cure the cut soap in a single layer, turning daily for 3 to 6 weeks. When properly cured the soap will be gentle and nondrying. Use within 1 year.

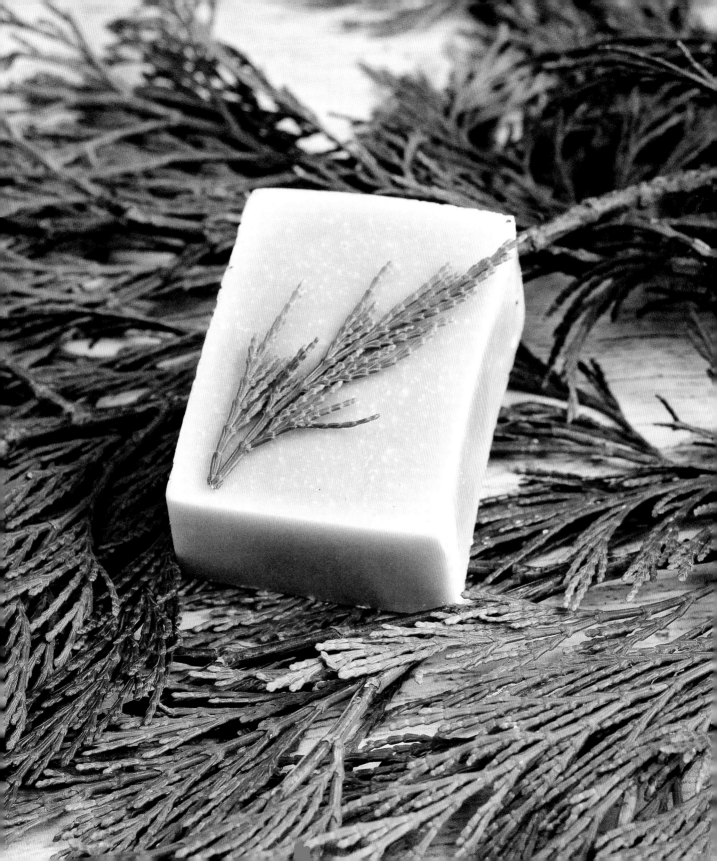

OREGON GRAPE

OTHER COMMON NAMES: holly grape, grapeholly, leatherleaf mahonia

LATIN NAME: *Mahonia aquifolium, M. repens, M. nervosa*

HERBAL ENERGETICS: cool/dry

THERAPEUTIC ACTIONS: alterative, anti-inflammatory, antimicrobial, antioxidant, astringent, cholagogue, diuretic, hepatic, hypoglycemic, immune-modulating, laxative, stimulant

PARTS USED: root

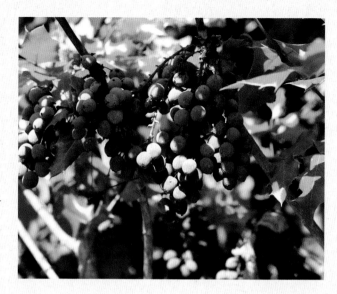

HERBAL MONOGRAPH

As a child I was always told that the berries of the enormous, holly-like bush outside my grandparents' house were poisonous. The attractive blue berries notwithstanding, I was sufficiently deterred by both the warning and the sharp-pointed, formidable leaves. A "look but don't touch" plant. That is until I learned of its medicinal value, and, shockingly, of its edibility. It's a "touch" plant now.

Oregon grape has such medicinal value that it is well worth the effort—and the pokes that one may endure—to harvest the precious golden roots and inner bark. Even the sour, bitter berries are incredibly tasty when creatively prepared. As one of the most antimicrobial agents in the plant world, Oregon grape puts the "anti" in antimicrobial, while also bringing a host of other healing benefits to the infection fight.

The woody yellow roots of Oregon grape are ripe with a constituent called berberine. Muscular berberine is a powerful antimicrobial agent capable of delivering a powerful punch to infections considered resistant to more conventional methods of treatment. Research indicates that berberine has an inhibitory effect on methicillin-resistant *Staphylococcus aureus*, and it also increases the efficacy of modern pharmaceutical treatments such as ampicillin and oxacillin. In the wake of antibiotic-resistant bacteria, Oregon grape holds promise as a botanical crusader against such infections. This botanical can be highly effective against respiratory and urinary tract complaints, most specifically when the complaint relates to the damp heat of these organ systems. Furthermore, there is some indication that it may be effective against *H. pylori*, a bacterium that contributes to digestive tract ulcerations and stomach cancer.

Oregon grape also has a strong affinity for the liver, benefitting hot, stagnant conditions. This herb addresses liver-related complaints such as dry, itchy skin, constipation, low metabolism and upset stomach with a sense of fullness in the upper abdomen. While addressing those symptoms, often lumped together as the product of a "sluggish" or "toxic" liver, Oregon grape is a specific herb for more acute concerns such as jaundice and hepatitis.

Where there is insufficient bile (observed with fatty stools and headache) or overproduction of bile (associated with diarrhea and unexplained weight loss), we find Oregon grape to be a great regulator, restoring good health to the gall bladder. By association with its gall bladder benefits, it also aids in digestion. There is also some clinical evidence demonstrating that the constituent berberine is as effective in treating type II diabetes as the more conventional treatment metformin. While it would take an absurdly high dose of Oregon grape root to achieve similar results, it stands to reason that a more traditional, reasonable dose of the herb would have a positive impact on blood glucose levels.

Perhaps one of the most exciting real-world applications of this botanical is for the treatment of chronic skin complaints such as acne, atopic dermatitis, eczema and psoriasis. Several different studies indicate that ointments prepared with Oregon grape as an ingredient helped to relieve these various complaints as well as or better than more conventional treatments. It would appear that the broad-spectrum antimicrobial and anti-inflammatory properties, as well as the profound benefits for the liver when taken internally, are at play here.

BEST PREPARATIONS: Oregon grape root can be tinctured either fresh or dried, and the dried roots can be used to infuse oils for the creation of ointments. The root is unquestionably bitter, but it can be consumed as a tea in concert with more hospitable, palatable herbs.

The berries, while quite unpalatable eaten out of hand, can produce fine jams, jellies and curds with a unique, feral flavor. I have even produced a lovely mead using Oregon grape berries that was very quaffable and capable of some bottle aging.

HERBAL SUBSTITUTES: Barberry (*Berberis vulgaris*): antimicrobial | goldenseal (*Hydrastis canadensis*): AT RISK. Avoid wild harvest of this herb.

SAFETY AND PRECAUTIONS

As a drying herb, Oregon grape may aggravate certain kidney and urinary conditions if taken incorrectly or excessively. Avoid if you have kidney disease. Oregon grape may also hasten the liver's processing of certain prescription medications that use the P450 pathway and should be avoided if taking those medications.

LOOK-ALIKES: Holly (*Ilex* spp.) TOXIC

IDENTIFY & GROW

🌸 **TYPE OF PLANT:** Evergreen shrub

🌸 **HABITAT:** Oregon grape is native to shady forested areas, with rich, loamy, moist but well-drained soils that have an acidic pH. However, Oregon grape is a well-adapted plant that is tolerant of full sun, so long as the soil is not arid or alkaline.

🌸 **HEIGHT:** 3–5' (1–1.5 m)

🌸 **LEAF:** Compound, pinnate, sharp, glossy, holly-like leaves in shades of green and burgundy arranged alternately

🌸 **ROOT:** Woody roots reveal a bright yellow interior when scrubbed gently of dirt

🌸 **FLOWER:** Clusters of bright yellow flowers appear mid-spring

🌸 **FRUIT:** Dusky blue round to slightly elongated berries appear mid- to late summer.

🌸 **GROWING INFORMATION:** Oregon grape is a common municipal plant due to its virtually maintenance-free existence. It makes a lovely landscape shrub as it has four seasons of interest, with the glossy green foliage

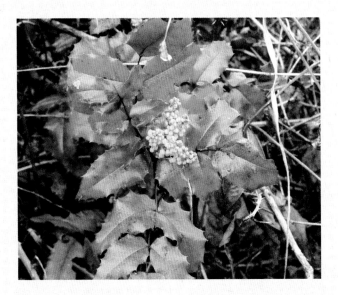

often blushing burgundy during the colder months of the year. Plant in areas protected from harsh winds or blazing sunlight. Oregon grape will prefer soils that are slightly acidic and moderately moisture retentive. Bonus: due to the prickly foliage, Oregon grape can make an outstanding theft deterrent when planted below windows or near access points of the home.

🌸 **FORAGE OR GROW?** I almost err toward the suggestion of growing this botanical. Although prolific in the Pacific Northwest, it is not as abundant in other regions and has officially made the "watch" list with the United Plant Savers. It makes an outstanding landscape shrub.

BEST HARVEST PRACTICES

EDIBLE BERRY HARVEST WINDOW: Mid-summer

ROOT HARVEST WINDOW: Early fall, after fruiting

To avoid killing an entire plant, the dirt can be scraped away from a larger plant's root system and the rootlets trimmed; replace the soil. Roots should be scrubbed and rinsed thoroughly, then chopped and dried. If foraging, be sure to only harvest roots from an area of substantial Oregon grape presence. Alternatively, the inner bark of smaller limbs also contains a considerable amount of berberine and can be used in place of roots, although their constituent profile is not quite as impressive. Beware, the leaves are very sharp. Wear gloves and long sleeves to protect yourself from painful pokes.

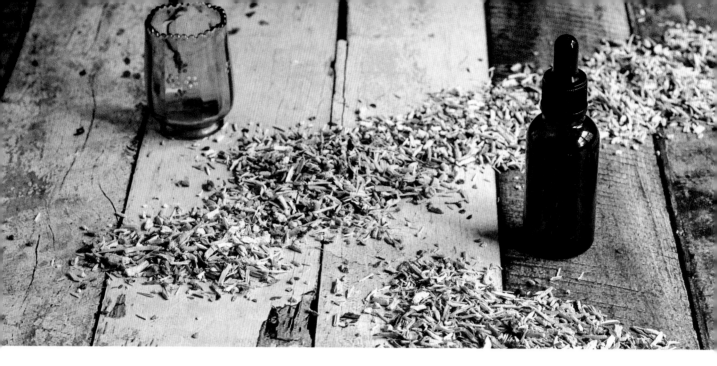

OREGON GRAPE ROOT TINCTURE FOR DIGESTIVE WELLNESS & INFECTION FIGHTING

This bitter little tincture is sure to rev your digestive juices into high gear. It is also a potent infection fighter. Take a little before meals or at the first sign of illness to support wellness.

YIELD: 1 pint (480 ml)

ADULT/TEEN DOSE: 1–2½ droppers full (1.5–4 ml), 3 times daily

CHILD'S DOSE, AGES 6–12: 1 dropper full (1.5 ml), 3 times daily

SMALL CHILD'S DOSE: 10–20 drops, 3 times daily

INGREDIENTS

2 cups (480 ml) 100 proof spirits (vodka recommended)

1½ cups (125 g) fresh Oregon grape root, chopped

INSTRUCTIONS

Combine the spirits and Oregon grape root in a jar with a tight-fitting lid. Infuse for a minimum of 6 weeks, shaking daily.

When the infusion is complete, strain the tincture through two layers of flour sack cloth into a liquid measuring cup. Pour into 1- or 2-ounce (30- or 60-ml) amber glass dropper bottles or into a pint-sized (480-ml) master amber glass bottle for dispensing. Keep in a cool, dry place. Use within 1 year.

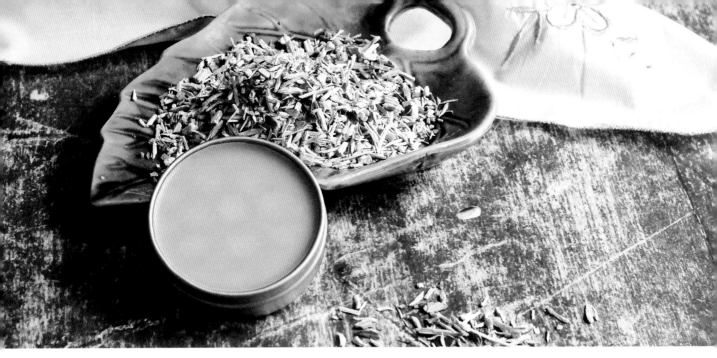

OREGON GRAPE OINTMENT FOR SCALY PATCHES & IRRITATED SKIN

This salve is a soothing balm for scaly, patchy skin conditions such as eczema, psoriasis and contact dermatitis. Regular use of this salve may help to reduce redness and uneven texture, and return the skin surface to good health.

YIELD: approximately 8 ounces (240 ml)

INGREDIENTS

½ cup (35 g) dried Oregon grape root

1 cup (240 ml) base oil blend of your choice (I like a blend of 50/50 olive oil to coconut oil)

2–4 tbsp (20–40 g) beeswax pastilles

INSTRUCTIONS

Using the regular or heated oil infusion method (page 12), infuse the Oregon grape into the base oils. After the oil is adequately infused, strain through muslin or cheese cloth.

Return the oil to a double boiler, add the beeswax and warm until completely melted. Remove the oil-beeswax mixture from the heat. Pour the salve into individual 2-ounce (60-ml) containers, approximately 4, or other similarly sized jars. Allow to cool completely before putting a lid on the container.

Apply to affected skin as needed. Use within 1 year.

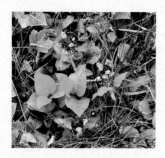

SELF HEAL

OTHER COMMON NAMES: heal-all, carpenter weed

LATIN NAME: *Prunella vulgaris*

HERBAL ENERGETICS: cool/neutral

THERAPEUTIC ACTIONS: antibacterial, antioxidant, antiseptic, antispasmodic, antiviral, astringent, carminative, demulcent, digestive, diuretic, febrifuge, hypotensive, immune-modulating, stimulant, styptic, tonic, vermifuge, vulnerary

PARTS USED: aerial parts

HERBAL MONOGRAPH

With a common name like self heal, one can expect that this is plant for a variety of complaints. But perhaps one of the attributes of this fine little herb that attracts me most is its proactiveness. Self heal is uniquely antioxidant in action, making it an excellent herb for protecting the skin from the damaging effects of UVA exposure. A 2006 study demonstrated a measurable reduction of the oxidative damage to skin cells with self heal extract, which offers great promise for botanical sun-care formulations. Additionally, as a cooling astringent, a simple water infusion cooled to room temperature and applied as a compress to a sunburn can bring immediate relief.

Self heal is yet another "wound herb" that can help to speed the healing of an injury or sore. Being styptic in nature, it may help to reduce blood loss from a minor wound and encourage the healthy and necessary scabbing process. It may also help to reduce scarring by reducing inflammation and countering infection in the wound. Additionally, this botanical is especially effective for viral sores such as shingles, HPV and fever blisters, making it one of the unique herbs capable of treating these difficult-to-address sores.

Self heal is especially soothing for painful inflammation of the throat and tonsils and is known to calm the immune-system response to seasonal allergies. It is also an excellent herb to consider for complaints of the digestive and urinary tracts. Self heal promotes the expulsion of internal parasites, relieves painful gas and bloating, cools inflammation of gut and urinary tract mucosa and tones lax intestinal and bladder tissues. It also promotes good blood pressure and soothes a hot fever.

BEST PREPARATIONS: Self heal is a pleasantly bitter herb with a flavor somewhat like rosemary, making for a palatable tea. For ulcers and abscesses about the mouth, tonsils and throat, a salt water gargle infused with dried self heal might offer lasting relief and speed healing. Base oils can be infused with the dried herb for an antioxidant-rich moisturizing oil.

HERBAL SUBSTITUTES: Yarrow (*Achillea millefolium*): styptic

SAFETY AND PRECAUTIONS

Self heal is considered safe for external use. There are no known contraindications for internal use, but if you are pregnant, nursing or taking prescription medication, please consult your physician before using this or any other herb.

LOOK-ALIKES: Purple dead-nettle (*Lamium purpureum*)

IDENTIFY & GROW

TYPE OF PLANT: Perennial

HABITAT: Self heal can often be found in meadows and at the edges of moist forests. It's a frequent "weed" in lawns and gardens in areas of dappled shade.

HEIGHT: 3–12" (8–30 cm)

LEAF: Small green, oval- to lance-shaped leaves arranged opposite on a central stem

STEM: Square

FLOWER: Lilac to purple flower spike tops stem mid-summer. Individual petals have a "lipped" appearance.

GROWING INFORMATION: Self heal seeds can be started indoors 8 to 10 weeks before the last frost and then transplanted to a moist and shady spot. As a member of the mint family, it divides easily and will quickly spread in its preferred environment.

FORAGE OR GROW? Self heal is easy to identify once it flowers. That fact, paired with its tendency to spread, makes me vote for self heal as an herb to forage for.

BEST HARVEST PRACTICES

FLOWERING TOP HARVEST WINDOW: Early to mid-summer

Self heal can be cut close to the ground frequently throughout the growing season to encourage new growth. It should be dried quickly to preserve its constituents.

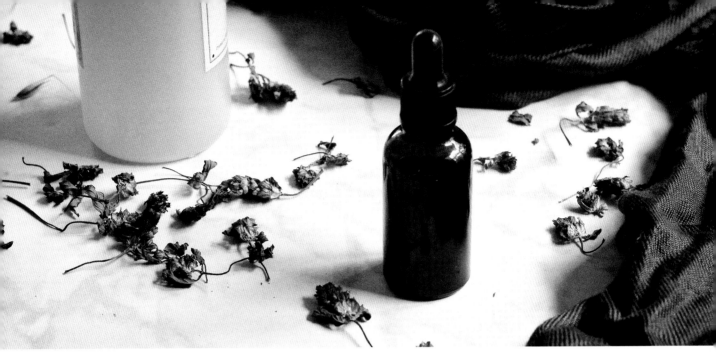

ANTIOXIDANT SELF HEAL DAY OIL

The outstanding antioxidant benefits of self heal make this lightweight moisturizing oil perfect for day use. Self heal provides an herbal barrier between environmental stressors and your skin, and gives you an additional layer of protection against the potentially damaging rays of the sun. Lightweight and nongreasy, this oil works well under makeup once fully absorbed. The optional carrot seed oil offers additional antioxidant action. Although this oil offers protection from oxidizing free radicals, it should not be considered a broad-spectrum sun screen.

Freshly picked self heal flowers can be wilted by laying them out in a single layer to dry for approximately 24 hours prior to infusion, which will help prevent spoilage with the fresh plant.

YIELD: approximately 8 ounces (240 ml)

INGREDIENTS

1 cup (240 ml) jojoba oil

½ cup (25 g) dried or wilted self heal

48 drops wild carrot seed essential oil (optional)

INSTRUCTIONS

Infuse the jojoba oil with the self heal using one of the infusion methods mentioned on page 12. When the infusion is complete, strain through two layers of flour sack cloth into a liquid measuring cup. If adding essential oil, do so at this time and stir well to combine. Pour into 1- or 2-ounce (30- or 60-ml) amber glass bottles.

To apply, add several drops into your palm and warm slightly with both hands before patting onto a clean, dry face. Allow the oil to absorb into skin before applying makeup. Use within 1 year.

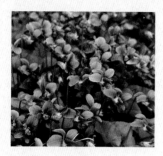

VIOLET

OTHER COMMON NAMES: viola, pansy, Johnny-jump-up, heartsease, kiss-me-at-the-gate

LATIN NAME: *Viola odorata, V. sororia, V. tricolor, V. papilionacea*
There are over 50 species with some degree of interchangeability.

HERBAL ENERGETICS: cool/moist

THERAPEUTIC ACTIONS: alterative, analgesic, anti-inflammatory, antiseptic, demulcent, diuretic, laxative, lymphatic, nervine, nutritive, purgative (roots and seeds), sedative, tonic

PARTS USED: leaf, flower

HERBAL MONOGRAPH

If there ever was a flower more fabled than the rose, it is most certainly the violet. As school children, violet entered our lexicon as "roses are red, violets are blue." It is often seen as a flower associated with Valentine's Day imagery, and some of its common names refer to stolen and secretive kisses. A Greek myth tells that Zeus provided a field of violets for his lover to graze after he turned her to a white heifer to save her from the jealous wrath of Hera. In Roman mythology, we learn that Venus beat a few fair maidens blue and turned them into violets upon her son Cupid's declaration that the maidens were more beautiful. Early Christians held that violets once pointed their countenance to the sky, but after the crucifixion, the flowers nodded to the ground in despair. In an interesting dichotomy, Christianity sees the flower as a symbol of modesty and humility, while more pagan cultures often associate violets with jealousy, sex and love/lust. Whatever the symbolism, violets are revered. Perhaps even greater than violet symbolism is the vast medicinal application of this precious botanical.

Although the fragrant "sweet violet" (*Viola odorata*) is most often touted in herbal repertories, there are many species of the *Viola* genus, known as "violets" and their associated common names—which are practically as abundant as the members of the violet family. Most can be used interchangeably; edibility and palatability may differ among the species. Some sources indicate that wild, yellow flowering species are "soapy" and undesirable due to a high saponin content. Yet, most common members of the *Viola* hold similar medicinal value—meaning that your cultivated potted plants may be just the remedy you are looking for, assuming that they are free of contamination.

Violets are the great soothers of the plant world, gently encouraging flow and movement of internal fluids. Most often the leaves and flowers are used in combination. This botanical is often used in cough remedies. Being demulcent and lymphatic, it is particularly useful for hot, dry conditions of the throat, coupled with hard, painful lymph glands under the jaw. I think of violets when there are complaints of pain and difficulty swallowing, irritable, dry cough and palpable nodules along the neck. Similarly, violets are often suggested to soothe ulcerations of the mouth and esophagus.

Chief among violet's many virtues is as a profound lymphatic. This is easily observed in the lymph tissues around the neck, but violet seems to have a particular affinity for the axillary (armpit to breast) and groin nodes as well. The lymphatic system does not have autonomous circulation, thus requiring movement and manual manipulation to circulate. Herbs such as violet are an excellent remedy to increase lymphatic drainage and soften hardened nodes. As it pertains to breast health, violet helps to soften fibrous breast tissue and cysts when combined with a gentle massage of concerning areas. Moreover, there is even some science to indicate that violet may have some anticancer potential. A 2014 study successfully demonstrated inhibition of activated lymphocyte cell proliferation using an aqueous *Viola tricolor* extract. Another 2017 study suggests that *Voila odorata* may have anti-melanogenic properties which show promise in the area of skin cancer research. While clearly these small studies do not constitute a "cancer cure," they do offer new and interesting potential for this botanical.

Violets are often overlooked as a nutritive tonic. They are abundant in vitamins A and C, rich in minerals and contain a phytonutrient known as rutin, which is associated with strengthening blood vessels—perhaps evidenced in the common name "heartsease." Violets, prepared with other alterative herbs such as chickweed, nettle and dock, will help the liver to purge excessive toxin buildup and recharge the batteries of a sluggish circulatory system.

Slightly sedative and analgesic and abundantly nervine, violets are often suggested when tension is associated with pain and irritability. Tradition suggests that violets placed about the head relieve headaches. Consumed as a tea with other nervine herbs, violet can promote calm and clarity, without making one overly sleepy.

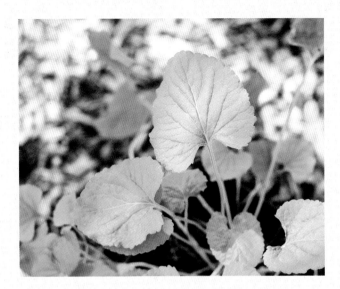

IDENTIFY & GROW

🌸 **TYPE OF PLANT**: Perennial (sometimes annual)

🌸 **HABITAT**: Violets prefer partial shade and moisture-retentive soils. They are generally found in wooded areas and shady lawns. In certain situations, violets may be spotted in sunnier locations, but they are intolerant of extreme heat and often wilt mid-summer in such areas. Cultivated varieties, frequently referred to as pansies, can be spotted in garden centers as early as late winter.

🌸 **HEIGHT**: 6–10" (15–25 cm)

🌸 **LEAF**: Simple, basal or alternate depending on species; palmate leaves with a "scalloped" margin, often heart-shaped to kidney bean–shaped

🌸 **STEM**: Flowers arise on leafless stalks

🌸 **FLOWER**: Violets appear most often in shades of blue-purple and variation on the theme such as white and blue stripes, although white and yellow wild varieties exist. All violets are irregular flowers with five petals, stamens and sepals each. Cultivated pansies can be splashier in color, often with yellow centers. Interestingly, the early spring flowers are sterile; it is a second, rather unnoticeable, flower that produces seed.

🌸 **SEED**: Seeds are mature in late summer to early fall in three-valved capsules.

🌸 **GROWING INFORMATION**: Violets grow well in moist, moderately shady areas. Violets can be propagated by root division or will often freely reseed when healthy and established.

🌸 **FORAGE OR GROW?** Violets are easy to grow and easy to identify. Even cultivated varieties have medicinal value. So, this one is a toss up. Forage and grow perhaps—one can.

BEST HARVEST PRACTICES
BEST FLOWER HARVEST WINDOW: Early spring

LEAF HARVEST WINDOW: Spring to summer

Harvesting flowers and leaves can be done easily with a pair of scissors, and the plant can benefit from a gentle harvest. Think of it like giving the violets a haircut. Do note that some native violet species are currently considered threatened and should not be harvested, especially when so many other options exist.

Violet is often called for when constipation with dry, hard stools is a complaint, due to the softening, lubricating effects of its mucilage, an insoluble fiber not unlike that of oatmeal. It is a gentle laxative that one can try before resorting to stronger herbs that often cause cramping. The seeds and roots of violet are thought to be purgative and emetic, so use with proper caution, if at all.

BEST PREPARATIONS: Violets lend themselves to a variety of preparations. Leaves and flowers are often dried and used in teas and infusions, ground to a paste for a poultice and tinctured in alcohol or vinegar. Vinegar is especially good for drawing out minerals and, when combined with honey, can be a tasty oxymel. Violets can be simmered with water and sugar to create a flavorful syrup that is perfect for relieving a cough or, mixed with sparkling water, for an herbal treat. Oils can also be infused with violets for salves, creams and massage bases.

Violets are also edible. The greens have a bland flavor somewhat similar to spinach and can be used in salad or even in soups where it acts as a milk-thickening agent. Violet flowers are very decorative, and they are often seen crystallized and topping worthy confections!

HERBAL SUBSTITUTES: Marshmallow (*Althea officinalis*): mucilage | blue vervain (*Verbena hastata*): tension

SAFETY AND PRECAUTIONS
Violets are largely considered safe, even while pregnant or nursing. Be advised that larger doses are purgative and laxative, so consume in reasonable amounts.

LOOK-ALIKES: Vinca (*Vinca* sp.), lesser celadine (*Ficaria verna*) TOXIC in large amounts

VIOLET SELF-CHECK CREAM FOR BREAST & LYMPHATIC HEALTH

One of the most vital actions a woman can take for her health is to preform regular breast exams. Vigilance leads to early detection and treatment of lumps and other abnormalities. This violet breast cream is designed for everyday use. That's right. I said every day. Applying this cream daily encourages familiarity with one's own breasts and how they may change and feel different throughout each cycle.

Violet promotes good lymphatic health and is thought to dissolve cystic tissue over time, and the rich oils included in the cream nourish and increase resiliency in the skin. This cream can also be used to address hardened lymph nodes in the underarm, groin and along the neck for both women and men.

If no essential oils are included in this blend, it is safe for nursing mamas and babies. Since this cream contains some water but no chemical preservative agent, it should be stored in the refrigerator between uses.

YIELD: approximately 2 ounces (60 ml)

INGREDIENTS

2 tbsp (6 g) dried violet leaf and flower, divided

8 oz (240 ml) water

2 tbsp (30 g) coconut oil or oil of your choice

1 tbsp (15 g) cocoa butter

1 tbsp (12 g) emulsifying wax pastilles

12 drops chamomile essential oil (optional)

INSTRUCTIONS

Make a violet infusion by infusing 1 tablespoon (3 g) of dried violet in 8 ounces (240 ml) of water just off the boil. Infuse for 20 minutes, then strain. Set aside 3 to 5 tablespoons (45 to 75 ml) of this infusion for the purposes of this recipe.

Using the double boiler method (page 12), infuse the coconut oil and cocoa butter with 1 tablespoon (3 g) of violet. Strain the infused oil through a fine-mesh sieve and return to the double boiler. Add the emulsifying wax and optional essential oil, and heat just until the wax is melted. Remove from the heat, and set aside. Meanwhile, adjust the temperature of the violet infusion to within about 10 degrees of the oils. In a small blender or with a handheld beater, slowly pour the reserved violet infusion into the oils to emulsify. Spoon or pipe into a 2-ounce (60-ml) container.

Apply using a sweeping motion from the underarm, around each breast and up the chest wall, and/or on the underarm, groin and neck. Use generously and make a new batch every 2 weeks. Refrigerate between uses.

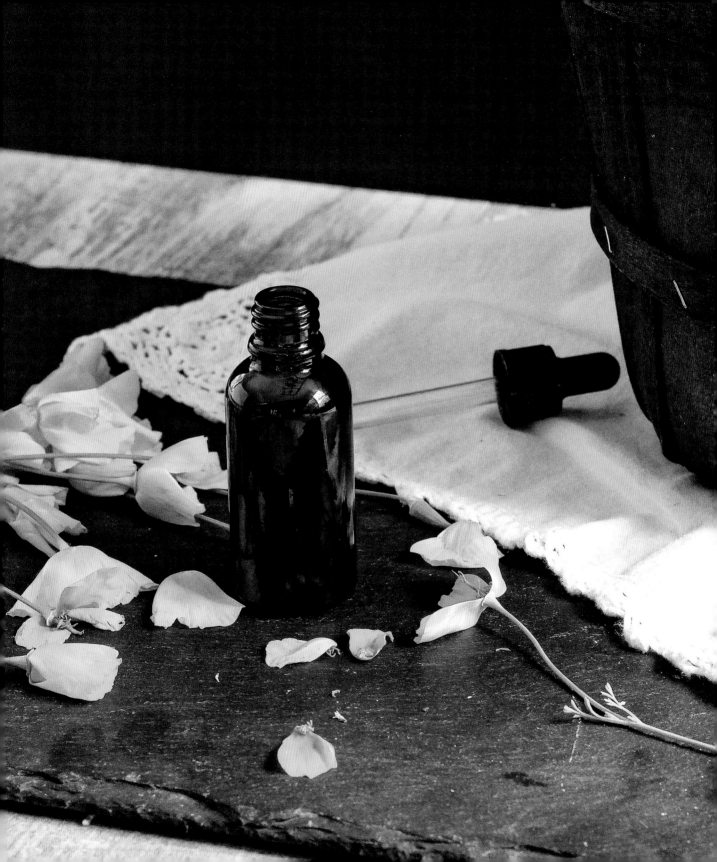

GRASSLAND SUN WORSHIPPERS TO REJUVENATE THE MIND AND BODY

THE GREAT GOLDEN STAR WANDERS its path through the sky each day, only to dip below the horizon each evening. Sun-worshipping botanicals bend and unfurl to capture every moment of the sun's warm embrace. Growing strong and bold under the great star's watchful eye, plants transform light and nutrients into beautiful medicine. From riotous wildflowers to more stoic hedgerows, sun-loving botanicals grace the landscape with their beauty and form.

Watch tall, immune-boosting echinacea sway gently in the breeze. Listen to the buzz of honey bees as they gather goodness from fields of sweet red clover, a cool, calming mineral-rich botanical. Draw in all the beauty and splendor that are the wild roses, the undisputed queen of flowers that blesses us with soft petals and vitamin C–rich flowers. Under the warming rays of the sun, all things are possible.

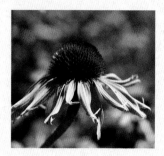

ECHINACEA

OTHER COMMON NAMES: coneflower, Sampson root, snakeroot

LATIN NAME: *Echinacea* spp. (*E. angustifolia* and *purpurea* are preferred in herbal medicine; *E. pallida* to a lesser extent)

HERBAL ENERGETICS: cool/dry

THERAPEUTIC ACTIONS: alterative, antibacterial, anti-inflammatory, antipyretic, antiseptic, antiviral, cardiovascular, immune-stimulator, lymphatic, sialagogue, vulnerary

PARTS USED: root, leaves, flowers

HERBAL MONOGRAPH

Nearly without fail I get one of four responses when I tell people I am an herbalist.

"Oh, so you work with weed." To which I respond that I do not work with marijuana, but I do work with botanicals commonly known as weeds.

"Cool. My sister sells essential oils, too." To which I respond that herbs and essential oils are different things and that I do not sell essential oils.

"So, you're a witch doctor." To which I respond, "No, I incorporate botanical medicine into holistic healthcare protocols using a combination of evidence-based and traditional folk research."

Or "Awesome, I take echinacea and haven't had a cold or flu in years." Bingo, this is somebody that is at least somewhat clued in and open to herbal medicine. But they still have a lot to learn. Banish echinacea to the cold and flu season, and you are missing a great many of its virtues.

While every response is clearly a teaching/learning opportunity, echinacea is the gateway herb for so many individuals into the world of botanical medicine. It is one of the few herbs that is in the lexicon of conventional, Western medicine. Its many benefits have secured its place in the cold and flu war chest. And echinacea offers so much more than just that.

To first address the elephant in the room: Echinacea is a profound immune system stimulant. It comes by its reputation rightfully. In a classic case of science catching up to what many traditional and folk herbalists already know, several important studies have found echinacea to be effective in shortening the duration of illness when taken at the onset of symptoms. A 2015 study of 473 individuals with influenza symptoms found echinacea to be as effective as the conventional influenza treatment, oseltamivir. A 2012 study suggests that certain standardized extracts of echinacea may be a suitable adjunct

to the "flu shot," demonstrating improved efficacy when used in conjunction. A four-month study of 755 individuals, split into echinacea prophylactic treatment and placebo, observed that the echinacea group experienced reduced common cold episodes, and those that did experience cold symptoms endured fewer episodic days compared to the placebo group. Researchers also noted that the echinacea group demonstrated no increased safety risk compared to the placebo group, and they suggested that echinacea be considered for long-term prophylactic care. These and many other studies confirm what herbalists have known for some time: echinacea makes for good cold and flu care. While the exact mechanism by which echinacea provides these benefits is currently unknown, it is thought that this herb helps to increase white blood cell count and promote phagocytosis—effectively scavenging viral and bacterial invaders.

While some evidence suggests that the herb may be a possible preventative, I tend to think of echinacea as the great rally-er and mobilizer of immunity "troops" to be used at the first sign of cold or flu, such as a runny nose, congestion, cough, fever or swollen lymph nodes.

With the cold and flu facet of echinacea well established, it is important to understand the other aspects of this herb that make it so very useful. We can turn our attention first to oral health. Echinacea is considered a sialagogue—that is, it induces the salivary response. And much like I deemed echinacea the gateway to herbal medicine, the mouth is the gateway to our body health. It is now becoming more generally understood that oral health plays an enormous role in the total body. In fact, several conditions such as endocarditis, cardiovascular disease, preterm birth and low birthweight have been linked to poor oral health. Furthermore, many conditions contribute to less than ideal oral conditions such as diabetes, osteoporosis, Alzheimer's and HIV/AIDS.

In many cases, it is "dry mouth" that upsets that natural bacterial balance, thereby opening the door to cavities, gum disease and other opportunistic infections. As a sialagogue, echinacea helps to restore saliva flow and promote healthier oral conditions.

In fact, in a study of intensive-care patients receiving tracheal intubation, researchers noted that the group receiving an echinacea mouthwash had decreased mouth microflora compared to the control group. The study concluded that echinacea mouthwash may be a preventative measure for ventilation-associated pneumonia. Traditionally, we use echinacea to address dry mouth, spongy gums and oral ulcerations. On a related note, increased salivary action plays an important role in the early stages of digestion, releasing the enzyme amylase, which helps to break down certain carbohydrates.

Echinacea is most often thought of as an internal herbal medicine, but it is an excellent topical first aid as well. Applied as a compress over poison oak/ivy rashes, echinacea can bring soothing relief. It is also a frontline defense for insect bites, as well as a bushcraft emergency remedy for venomous snake bites. A poultice of leaves and flowers applied to the stricken area and tincture taken internally are thought to delay sepsis and stop the spread of the venom while immediate medical attention is sought.

BEST PREPARATIONS: Echinacea can be prepared for a variety of internal and external applications. The root, as well as the aerial parts, can be tinctured fresh or dried. Fresh poultices consisting of leaves and flowers can easily be applied to the affected area. A strong infusion of the herb (roots or aerial parts) can be prepared and applied to rashes and skin irritations as a compress. Teas and mouthwashes prepared from the whole plant are also an excellent way of using this herb.

Echinacea flowers are edible and can be used fresh for salads and as decoration for baked goods.

Echinacea preparations are best taken at the onset of symptoms rather than as a "preventative solution."

HERBAL SUBSTITUTES: Elderberry (*Sambucus* spp.): immunity | astragalus (*Astragalus membranaceus*): immunity

SAFETY AND PRECAUTIONS
If you are pregnant, nursing or taking prescription medication, please consult your physician before taking this or any other herb. Echinacea may not be safe for those with autoimmune disorders. Avoid if you are allergic to members of the *Asteraceae* (daisy) family.

LOOK-ALIKES: Daisy (*Bellis* sp.), black-eyed susan (*Rudbeckia hirta*)

IDENTIFY & GROW
TYPE OF PLANT: Perennial

HABITAT: This is an upright, drought-tolerant, sun-loving herbaceous plant that thrives in moderately rich, well-drained soils. Prefers prairie-like conditions.

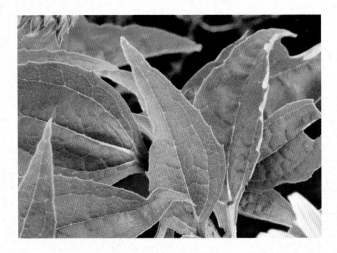

HEIGHT: 2–4' (0.6–1.2 m)

LEAF: Elongated, ovoid or narrow leaf. Spring growth starts as a basal clump, but leaves arrange alternately as the season progresses. Depending on the particular species, leaves may or may not be serrated.

STEM: Hairy

FLOWER: Large composite flowers with central cone in shades of pink, mauve and occasionally ivory

GROWING INFORMATION: To ensure good seed germination, seeds should be cold stratified. To cold stratify echinacea seeds, sow them directly in the fall, or soak in water, strain, wrap in a paper towel or newsprint and store in the refrigerator for up to 10 weeks. Plant seeds or seedlings in full sun in pH neutral soil. While echinacea will thrive in nutrient dense soils, avoid overuse of fertilizer or organic material as this will promote "leggy" plants and sprawling habit.

FORAGE OR GROW? Native prairies of echinacea have been ravaged by overzealous wildcrafters and the herbal supplement industry. This is an herb to grow.

BEST HARVEST PRACTICES
LEAF AND FLOWER HARVEST WINDOW: Summer

ROOT HARVEST WINDOW: Fall

Leaves and flowers can be collected by shearing top growth throughout the growing season. In fact, this often promotes return bloom. Well-established roots can be collected in the fall, then cleaned and dried for storage or tinctured fresh. If preparing a whole plant tincture (page 54), you can harvest the whole plant at peak flowering.

ECHINACEA IMMUNITY SYRUP

Echinacea is one of the most popular herbal remedies used today. While there are some great products and recipes available, I often feel that many circumvent a very important action. When we use encapsulated herbs, and, to some extent, tinctures, herbs don't spend a lot of time in our mouths. But it is in our mouths that echinacea provides a great deal of its medicine value via the promotion of saliva. When we have a good oral environment and moisture balance in our mouths, we become far less susceptible to infection.

This tasty syrup is best taken when you know that you have been exposed to cold or flu, or at the first sign of symptoms. The additions of lemon balm and lemon zest offer bright, citrusy flavor and vitamin C.

YIELD: 1 generous pint (480+ ml)

ADULT DOSE, AGES 12 AND UP: 1 tablespoon (15 ml), every 4 to 6 hours

CHILD'S DOSE, AGES 6–11: 1–2 teaspoons (5–10 ml), every 4 to 6 hours

CHILD'S DOSE, AGES 2–5: ¼–½ teaspoon, every 4 to 6 hours

INGREDIENTS

2 cups (480 ml) water

2 cups (500 g) raw organic sugar

½ cup (33 g) dried echinacea root

Zest of 1 lemon

½ cup (12 g) dried lemon balm

INSTRUCTIONS

In a small saucepan, add the water, sugar, echinacea root and lemon zest. Over medium heat, bring the mixture to a simmer. Gently simmer for approximately 5 minutes, or until the mixture is slightly reduced and thickened to a thin syrup. Remove from the heat, and stir in the lemon balm. Cool completely.

When the syrup is cooled, strain through a fine-mesh sieve into a liquid measuring cup. Pour into a glass bottle or jar, and store in the refrigerator. Use within 1 month.

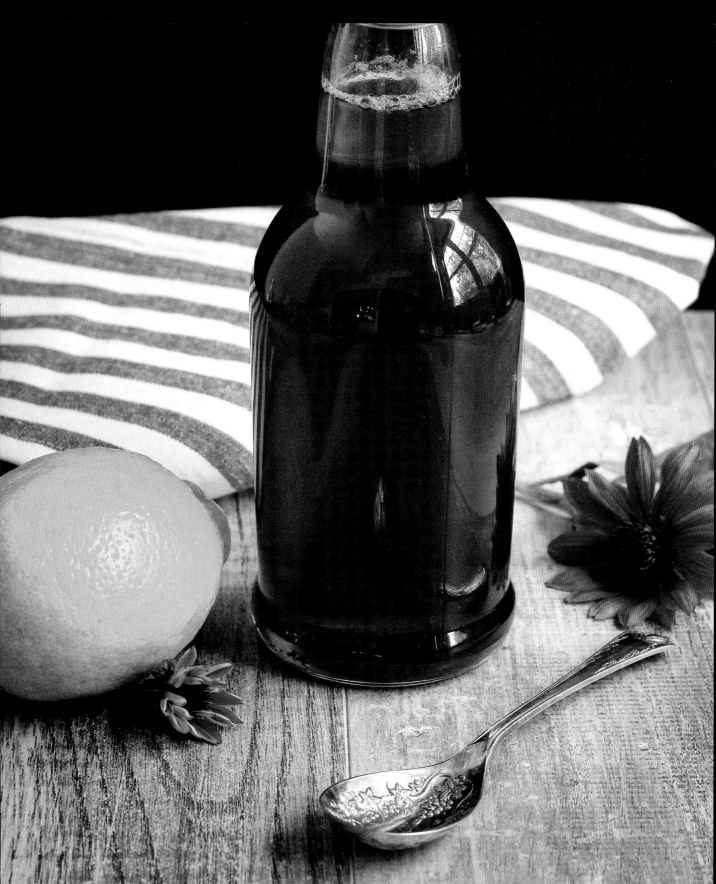

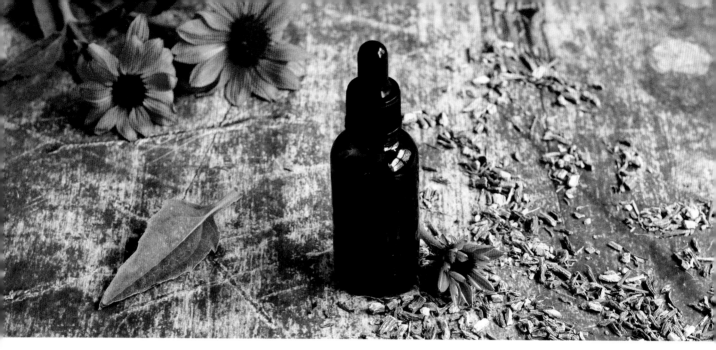

ECHINACEA WHOLE PLANT TINCTURE

Although echinacea root traditionally gets the most attention for its medicinal benefits, herbalists are increasingly advocating for whole plant use. Including leaves and flowers along with the root ensures your tincture is rich in immune-boosting constituents!

From a conservation standpoint, I particularly love the "whole plant concept." Instead of gathering roots from a multitude of plants in order to have enough plant material, one plant would provide more than enough root, leaf and flower for this recipe! Harvest the whole plant during peak flowering, washing the roots thoroughly before preparing the tincture. This tincture should be taken at the first sign of cold and flu symptoms. It can also be used as a gargle or mouthwash in water for oral health.

YIELD: 1 pint (480 ml)

ADULT DOSE: 1–3 droppers full (1.5–4.5 ml), 3 times daily

CHILD'S DOSE, AGES 6–12: ½–1 dropper full (0.75–1.5 ml), 3 times daily

SMALL CHILD'S DOSE, AGES 2–5: 10–15 drops, 3 times daily

INGREDIENTS

2 cups (480 ml) 100 proof spirits (vodka recommended)

½ cup (65 g) fresh echinacea root, chopped

½ cup (25 g) fresh echinacea leaves, chopped

½ cup (25 g) fresh echinacea flowers, chopped

INSTRUCTIONS

Combine the spirits and echinacea root, leaves and flowers in a jar with a tight-fitting lid. Infuse for a minimum of 6 weeks, shaking daily. When the infusion is complete, strain the tincture through two layers of flour sack cloth into a liquid measuring cup. Pour into 1- or 2-ounce (30- or 60-ml) amber glass dropper bottles or into a pint-sized (480-ml) master amber glass bottle for dispensing. Use within 1 year.

YARROW

OTHER COMMON NAMES: milfoil, woundwort, soldier's wort, sanguinary

LATIN NAME: *Achillea millefolium*

HERBAL ENERGETICS: cool/dry

THERAPEUTIC ACTIONS: anodyne, anti-inflammatory, antimicrobial (bacteriostatic–Wood), antispasmodic, astringent, diaphoretic, digestive, diuretic, febrifuge, hepatic, hypotensive, styptic, vulnerary

PARTS USED: leaf and flower

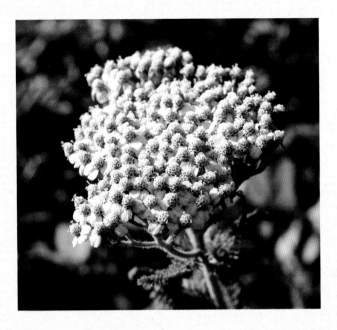

HERBAL MONOGRAPH

If somebody told me that I could only pick ten herbs for my apothecary . . . I would probably wilt from the stress of narrowing down my beloved herbs. Now if the same person then told me I could only pick one herb, then the task would get simpler.

I would pick yarrow.

Yarrow wins the prize for "most useful herb" in my book. Simply put, it is a workhorse. Offering a host of therapeutic actions, yarrow runs the gamut. It is a first aid herb. A digestive herb. An herb for women's reproductive health. An herb for fever. There is practically nothing that dear yarrow cannot do. Then add that it's a pretty, carefree perennial. It is in no way threatened or endangered. It's easy to harvest and process, and it's relatively palatable. Yarrow puts a checkmark in all the boxes.

Yarrow serves as my first choice "first aid" herb due to its styptic and antimicrobial properties. With its Latin name nodding to the great Greek hero Achilles, yarrow plays an important role in certain versions of the myth: his mother dipping him in a yarrow infusion while holding his heels, leaving that one spot as his only vulnerability.

Beyond the great myth, yarrow has long been considered a battleground herb, with many of its lesser-known names referring to soldiers, military and wounds. It simply has a profound and immeasurable ability to staunch the flow of blood from minor and even serious wounds. I, too, have found it to be a remarkable herb to stop the flow of blood after a grievous food processor wound on the eve of a holiday feast for which I was the hostess. From war wounds to kitchen mishaps, yarrow is my herb of choice. It is a fast and effective herbal remedy to bridge the gap while seeking medical attention (if necessary).

Not surprisingly, yarrow is also a plant ally to women's health. Yarrow is thought to act as a "pelvic decongestant," draining boggy and stagnant tissue, while stimulating blood flow. Herbalists use this botanical to help regulate menstrual flow, by both moderating excessive flow and stimulating delayed and scanty menses. It is particularly useful when there are complaints of uterine fibroids, ovarian cysts, endometriosis and cramping. Yarrow is also considered an excellent herb for addressing urinary tract infections, weak bladder and painful urination.

Yarrow is classified as a bitter herb—though it is not unpleasantly so, in my opinion. It has a flavor not unlike chamomile, but a bit more "green." As such, it is an herb that promotes good digestion by stimulating the flow of gastric juices. Cooling in its energetic properties, yarrow also may provide some relief for heartburn sufferers. It is also an herb to consider when bleeding ulcers are a concern.

Yarrow offers pain-relieving and inflammation-reducing properties, making it an excellent herb to address skin complaints such as sunburn, bug bites and rash. It is considered a minor bug repellant and a hair follicle stimulant. It is a gentle fever reducer, best suited for those that are red-skinned and hot to the touch, perhaps also complaining of no appetite and nausea.

BEST PREPARATIONS: Yarrow offers a broad selection of therapeutic actions and possible preparations. Dried yarrow can be powdered for a lightweight addition to any herbal first aid bag. Tincturing the fresh herb in witch hazel offers another wound treatment option. The fresh herb can be tinctured in alcohol for internal use. The dried herb is perfect for teas and infusions, as well as for infusing a base oil for salve-making purposes.

HERBAL SUBSTITUTES: Shepherd's purse (*Capsella bursa-pastoris*): styptic | calendula (*Calendula officinalis*): vulnerary

SAFETY AND PRECAUTIONS
Avoid yarrow internally if you are pregnant, nursing, taking prescription medication or have an allergy to members of the *Asteraceae* family.

LOOK-ALIKES: Queen Anne's lace (*Daucus carota*) | poison hemlock (*Conium maculatum*) EXTREMELY TOXIC

IDENTIFY & GROW

TYPE OF PLANT: Perennial

HABITAT: Yarrow is often found in light and well-drained soils, sometimes in rocky areas and outcroppings situated in full sun. As the flower heads can become quite large and heavy, yarrow may naturally appear in areas somewhat protected from the wind.

HEIGHT: 1–3' (0.3–1 m)

LEAF: 3–4" (8–10-cm) alternate, feathery leaves in blue-gray shades of green

STEM: Rough and angular

FLOWER: Large flattish cymes of tiny flowers resembling very small daisies. Traditionally, herbalists consider white flowering yarrow to have the most medicinal value, followed by the pink flowering cultivars, which are thought to have some emotional and spiritual well-being benefits. Sources seem unclear whether the yellow cultivars are medicinally valuable.

GROWING INFORMATION: Start yarrow seeds indoors 6 to 8 weeks before the last frost in spring. Transplant hardened off seedlings into a well-drained bed with plenty of compost in full sun. Give yarrow plenty of room to spread and protection from aggressive wind.

FORAGE OR GROW? Yarrow grows nearly everywhere in the world where the temperatures are moderate, and it is easily identifiable, making it a great foraging choice. Yarrow is an exceptional garden plant, known as the "plant doctor." It deters pests, increases nutrient availability, attracts pollinators and naturally increases the essential oil content of nearby plants. I vote that yarrow is an herb to grow.

BEST HARVEST PRACTICES
FLOWER AND LEAF HARVEST WINDOW: Mid-summer

Harvest long stems of yarrow leaves and flowers when the flowers are fully opened but not yet drying out. Separate flower tops and leaves on drying screens or hang to dry.

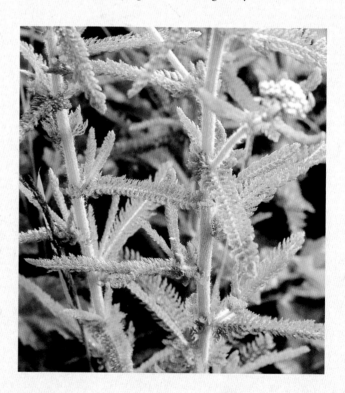

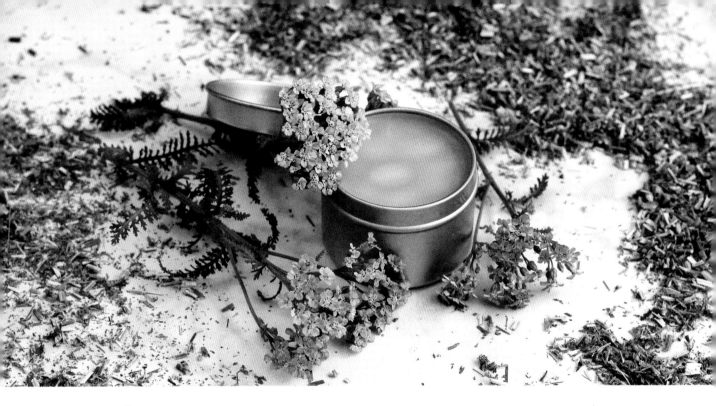

YARROW ALL-PURPOSE WOUND SALVE

This is a wound salve for all your scrapes, minor cuts and abrasions. Yarrow fights away infection-causing germs, slows bleeding from oozy wounds and encourages rapid wound closure. It is the best stuff around!

YIELD: approximately 8 ounces (240 ml)

INGREDIENTS

½ cup (25 g) dried yarrow leaf and flower

1 cup (240 ml) base oil blend of your choice (I like coconut oil and olive oil)

2–4 tbsp (20–40 g) beeswax pastilles

INSTRUCTIONS

Using the regular or heated oil infusion method (page 12), infuse the yarrow into the base oils. After the oil is adequately infused, strain through muslin or cheese cloth.

Return the oil to a double boiler, add the beeswax and warm until completely melted. Remove the oil-beeswax mixture from the heat. Pour into individual 2-ounce (60-ml) containers, approximately 4, or other similarly sized jars. Allow to cool completely before putting a lid on the container. Use within 1 year.

Apply as needed to minor cuts, scrapes and other injuries.

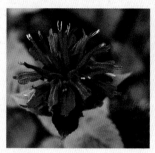
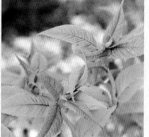

BEE BALM

OTHER COMMON NAMES: Oswego tea, bergamot

LATIN NAME: *Monarda* sp.

HERBAL ENERGETICS: warm/cool/dry

THERAPEUTIC ACTIONS: antibacterial, antifungal, antiseptic, antispasmodic, carminative, diaphoretic, diffusive, emmenagogue, nervine, relaxant, stimulant

PARTS USED: leaves and flowering tops

HERBAL MONOGRAPH

Some botanicals have really "got it going on." Tall, elegant and topped in shades of red, pink and purple, bee balm simply exudes beauty and confidence. She is no botanical wallflower.

And she isn't a medicinal wallflower either. Bee balm stimulates and invigorates, clearing boggy, fluid-filled tissues and cavities. It is an herb that I reach for anytime there are complaints of the upper respiratory system. It is particularly useful for stubborn sinus congestion and post nasal drip. Bee balm is a wonderful herb to use when there is a fever accompanied by cold, clammy skin, as well as wet, heavy coughs. Bee balm is particularly soothing to nausea caused by sinus drainage and is encouraging to a reticent appetite. It can also ameliorate bloating and gas, colic and nervous stomachs/diarrhea and can be useful for inflammation and infection in the intestinal tract. Bee balm is indicated for matters of candida overgrowth and "leaky gut syndrome."

The complex energetic nature and antiseptic qualities of bee balm also make it an excellent herb for the urinary tract and women's sexual health. Bee balm may calm bladder discomfort and inflammation of the urethra. It is also a first choice herb for addressing vaginal yeast infections, as well as helping to restore vaginal tone and sensation.

BEST PREPARATIONS: As teas and infusions, bee balm is excellent for lower respiratory, urinary and digestive complaints. Sitz baths and herbal douches provide relief for women's complaints. It also lends itself well to herbal steam to address upper respiratory congestion, and an herbal plaster or poultice can warm and invigorate a stodgy wet chest.

HERBAL SUBSTITUTES: Oregano (*Origanum vulgare*): antiseptic | thyme (*Thymus vulgaris*): antiseptic

SAFETY AND PRECAUTIONS

Avoid bee balm if you are pregnant or nursing.

LOOK-ALIKES: Members of the mint (Labiate) family due to foliage similarities, especially oregano due to scent

IDENTIFY & GROW

TYPE OF PLANT: Perennial

HABITAT: Native to North America, bee balm grows well in full sun to light shade. It prefers well-drained soils; some cultivars are more tolerant of boggier soils.

HEIGHT: 3–5' (1–1.5 m)

LEAF: Leaves are arranged opposite, and are lance-shaped with serrated margins. Foliage comes in various shades of green, sometimes with red- or rust-colored tinges.

STEM: Square

FLOWER: Flowers are best described as "firework-like" with many petals unfurling from the center out, in shades of pink, purple and red. They are highly attractive to pollinators such as bees and hummingbirds.

GROWING INFORMATION: Bee balm seeds can be directly sown in the fall or early spring before the last frost. Keep soil evenly moist during establishment. Bee balm is a good candidate for propagating via cutting and plants should be divided every three years. Cut flowers or deadhead to encourage repeat bloom throughout the summer.

FORAGE OR GROW? This North American native can be found in virtually every state or province on the continent. It is a favorite perennial in many garden centers and makes a very attractive landscape plant. My vote is that you add bee balm to your garden.

BEST HARVEST PRACTICES

FLOWER AND LEAF HARVEST WINDOW: Summer

Harvest flowering tops and leaves throughout the blooming period when the flowers are fully opened. Dry quickly.

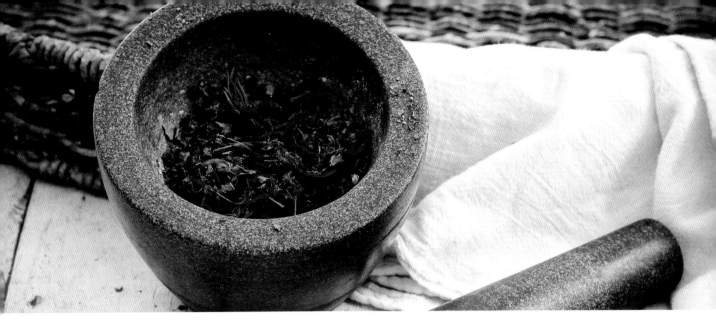

BEE BALM HERBAL PLASTER FOR BOGGY CHESTS & MURKY SINUSES

Picture this. It's late January. Your kids have been trading sniffles and colds with their classmates since last fall. Your immune system threw up its hands in defeat a week ago. Your sinuses are drippy, and there is an invisible elephant on your chest. You're sick and tired of being sick and tired, but you're not sick enough to get medical attention. Bee balm to the rescue! This chest plaster whipped up with dried, powdered herbs and a little flour and water, placed on the chest with a hot water bottle or heating pad will help to break up stubborn congestion and warm a soggy, winter-worn chest. This remedy is safe for children, although you may want to cut the quantities called for in half due to the reduced surface area of a child's chest.

YIELD: 1 application

INGREDIENTS

1 cup (25 g) dried bee balm leaves and flowers, ground to a powder

2 tbsp (15 g) all-purpose flour

Warm water, to make a spreadable paste

INSTRUCTIONS

Using a mortar and pestle or a dedicated coffee grinder, powder the bee balm until fine. In a small bowl, mix the powdered bee balm with the flour. Add enough warm water to make a spreadable paste. Apply the paste in a thin layer over the chest. Cover with a soft towel or a flour sack cloth, then place a hot water bottle or heating pad at its lowest setting on top of the cloth.

Lie on your back with the plaster on your chest and heating instrument in place for 20 to 30 minutes, while concentrating on taking deep, belly-filling breaths. Unlike mustard plasters that can be similarly applied, bee balm is far gentler, and no skin irritation is to be expected. However, if discomfort or a burning sensation is experienced, wash off the plaster immediately. After you're done resting with the plaster in place, wash the area with soap and water, then pat dry.

JAPANESE KNOTWEED

OTHER COMMON NAMES: donkey rhubarb, Japanese bamboo

LATIN NAME: *Fallopia japonica*

HERBAL ENERGETICS: cold/dry

THERAPEUTIC ACTIONS: analgesic, antibacterial, anti-inflammatory, antioxidant, antispirochetal, astringent, cardiovascular, diuretic, expectorant, immune stimulant, laxative, styptic

PARTS USED: root, early shoots (edible)

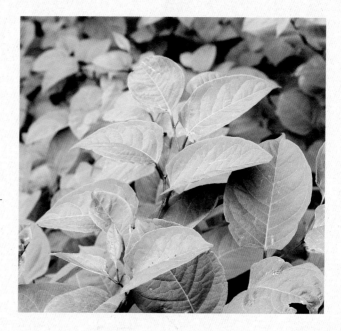

HERBAL MONOGRAPH

Few medicinal plants are reviled as much as Japanese knotweed. Despite its attractive appearance, Japanese knotweed is the scourge of farmers, gardeners, landscapers and ecologists alike. In its native land, knotweed is held in check by predation, but beyond eastern Asia, this botanical declares open season on native habitats. Records indicate knotweed's arrival in Europe may date as far back as 1825, and it is officially the botanical "persona non grata" throughout the United Kingdom, destroying native habitats and wreaking havoc on property values. Lest you think the U.K. is the only victim of knotweed's aggression, many other areas of Europe, North America and other areas of introduction are experiencing similar botanical assault. This plant resists eradication with virtually unparalleled tenacity. It is resistant to herbicides and physical removal—even the tiniest portion of root left in the soil can give rise to a new patch.

My own experience with knotweed in the landscape was first finding it flourishing along a fence line near an outbuilding at a former property. It had developed such a ferocious root system that it had actually cracked the cement slab and grown up and into the nearby building. We allowed our sheep to graze the early spring growth which did seem to greatly curtail its spread. Upon clearing invasive blackberries from an area of our current homestead, I laughed the most defeated cackle to find knotweed underneath. The irony of finding one invasive plant hiding under another did not escape me.

All this nastiness aside, Japanese knotweed is not without value. While it is most certainly not a botanical to plant outside its native habitat, it is a prime candidate for foraging. In fact, it is a highly medicinal plant that treats a very underserved part of the population. It addresses Lyme disease. Knotweed is among relatively few herbs that are effective against the spirochetal bacteria that cause Lyme disease and some of its coinfections, while also reducing the severity of symptoms. As part of the disease course, the bacteria initiate an inflammatory cascade; knotweed constituents inhibit these pathways, helping to alter the course of the disease. Additionally, this herb increases circulation to certain areas of the body that tend to harbor these infections, such as the skin, joints, heart and eyes. As such, Japanese knotweed is gaining popularity as a concurrent treatment beside modern antibiotics.

Beyond its possible implications in the fight against Lyme disease, Japanese knotweed offers a variety of other therapeutic actions. It regulates bowel function and diaphoresis, reduces blood loss, decreases water retention and dries wet, heavy chest conditions. Perhaps most interestingly, knotweed contains a great quantity of resveratrol: the constituent most closely associated with red wine and its cardiovascular benefit. Studies show that this botanical minimizes pro-inflammatory bio-markers and greatly reduces inflammation, thus supporting cardiovascular health.

BEST PREPARATIONS: The most effective means of extracting the important constituents of Japanese knotweed appear to be as a tincture.

Newly emerged Japanese knotweed stalks are a nutritious early spring food with a flavor similar to rhubarb. It is best prepared as sweet-tar pickle or chutney.

HERBAL SUBSTITUTES: Teasel (*Dipsacus fullonum*): Lyme disease | hawthorn (*Crataegus* sp.): cardiovascular

SAFETY AND PRECAUTIONS

Do not use Japanese knotweed concurrently with blood thinners. If you are suffering with Lyme disease, please consult a physician and disclose use of knotweed if applicable. If you are pregnant, nursing or taking prescription medication, please consult a physician before using this or any other herb.

LOOK-ALIKES: Pheasant berry (*Leycesteria formosa*), bamboo (*Bambuseae* sp.)

IDENTIFY & GROW

🌸 **TYPE OF PLANT:** Perennial

🌸 **HABITAT:** True to its highly invasive form, Japanese knotweed thrives in full sun, but will tolerate a fair amount of shade and can quickly spread in areas of disturbed soils. This plant will quickly choke out other vegetation and form large clumping hedges if not controlled.

🌸 **HEIGHT:** 3–10' (1–3 m)

🌸 **LEAF:** New leaf growth is rolled and burgundy-red, maturing to a green, heart-shaped leaf, arranged alternately on a bamboo-like stem.

🌸 **STEM:** Hollow, segment green stem with burgundy speckles; grows at the rate of almost 1 inch (2.5 cm) a day

🌸 **FLOWER:** Spikes of tiny creamy white flowers appear in late summer.

🌸 **ROOT:** Rhizomes have a dark exterior and an orange interior.

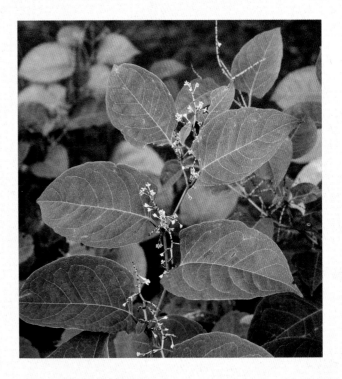

🌸 **GROWING INFORMATION: Do not grow Japanese knotweed outside of its native habitat in eastern Asia.** This highly invasive botanical even exhibits strong allelopathic tendencies—emitting toxins to nearby plant matter.

🌸 **FORAGE OR GROW?** This is DEFINITELY a botanical to forage. However, harvest only from areas that you know to be 100 percent spray-free as herbicide eradication takes frequent, repeated applications and even then it is highly unlikely to greatly mitigate its spread.

BEST HARVEST PRACTICES
ROOT HARVEST WINDOW: Fall

Roots are ideally lifted yearly in fall and promptly cleaned, sliced and tinctured. When possible, remove all traces of knotweed in an effort to control its spread.

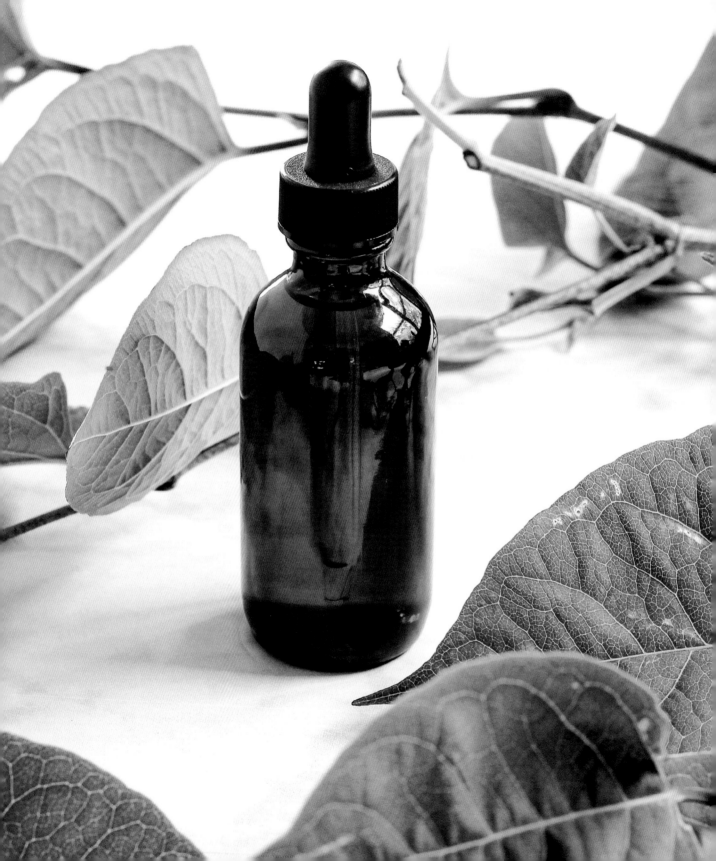

JAPANESE KNOTWEED TINCTURE FOR LYME DISEASE SUPPORT

While we could never realistically hope to eradicate this pesky invasive from its nonnative environments, making medicinal remedies from Japanese knotweed makes good use of this nuisance botanical. This is a great example of how herbal medicine can contribute to a more balanced ecosystem!

This tincture can be used as part of a holistic Lyme disease protocol to help rebuild the immune system and reduce the primary infection and coinfection levels.

YIELD: 1 pint (480 ml)

ADULT DOSE: ½–1 dropper full (0.75–1.5 ml), 3 times daily

CHILD'S DOSE, AGES 6–12: 10–15 drops, 3 times daily

CHILD'S DOSE, AGES 2–6: up to 5 drops, 3 times daily

INGREDIENTS

2 cups (480 ml) 100 proof spirits (vodka recommended)

1½ cups (180 g) fresh Japanese knotweed root, chopped

INSTRUCTIONS

Combine the spirits and Japanese knotweed root in a jar with a tight-fitting lid. Infuse for a minimum of 6 weeks, shaking daily.

When the infusion is complete, strain the tincture through two layers of flour sack cloth into a liquid measuring cup. Pour into 1- or 2-ounce (30- or 60-ml) amber glass dropper bottles or into a pint-sized (480-ml) master amber glass bottle for dispensing. Use within 1 year.

> **TIP:** If one has objections to using alcohol, a glycerin-based tincture can be prepared using the above recipe, substituting the glycerin for the alcohol. Follow the same general dosage guidelines, leaning toward the higher end of the dosage range recommended.

MULLEIN

OTHER COMMON NAMES: Aaron's rod, flannel leaf, Jacob's staff, Jupiter's staff

LATIN NAME: *Verbascum thapsus, V. olympicum*

HERBAL ENERGETICS: cool/neutral

THERAPEUTIC ACTIONS: anodyne (flower), anti-inflammatory, antispasmodic, astringent (root), demulcent (leaf), expectorant, lymphatic, vulnerary

PARTS USED: flowers, leaves, roots

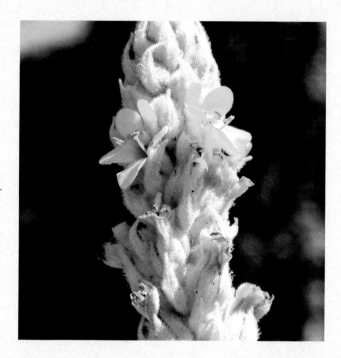

HERBAL MONOGRAPH

Mullein is one of those herbs that bridges the gap between armchair herbalism and more intense herbal learning. Mullein has some very practical medicinal applications, but it also offers us a unique view into some far more esoteric herbal concepts. It is an herb that teaches us so much about its benefits if we are just willing to learn from the plant itself. It is an herb that encourages us to follow our intuition. From its small fuzzy hairs to its tall, upright stature, mullein is a great herbal teacher.

I was first introduced to mullein with mullein flower ear oil (usually seen with garlic). Quite fitting, mullein flowers have an affinity for complaints of the head, more specifically the ears. Mullein flowers have exceptional pain and inflammation relieving qualities, making oil infused with the botanical extremely soothing to inflamed and irritated tissue. This is especially wonderful for childhood ear infections as modern antibiotics seem to show little to no difference in the duration and severity of infection. I also find mullein flower ear oil to be helpful when there seems to be residual sinus pressure on the ears. I have even found it to be useful for vertigo caused by inner ear fluid and pressure.

As we move down the mullein stalk, we are greeted by the fuzzy, flannel-like leaves. The soft downy hairs remind me of cilia, the hair-like organelles that cover parts of the respiratory tract. It is quite appropriate that mullein leaves are a strong respiratory ally. Mullein is thought to nourish cilia and support cilia function when there is a history of inhaled irritants and smoking. It is a very useful herb for dry, hot coughs that are accompanied by rib pain and tenderness. Herbalists reach for mullein for chronic respiratory concerns such as low-grade persistent bronchitis, but it is also helpful for more acute concerns such as pneumonia. Mullein is even used as a tobacco substitute for smoking cessation and to deliver the antispasmodic benefits deep into the lungs in an expedient manner.

Mullein leaves don't only aid the respiratory system. The lower leaves, along with the root, are considered for all matters of low back pain and strain. It is thought that the tall, erect stature and the plant's resilience to wind damage represents its ability to strengthen and support connective tissues.

BEST PREPARATIONS: Mullein is a versatile herb both medicinally and in its various preparations. Dried mullein flowers can be infused into base oils—traditionally with garlic to act as an antiseptic—for ear complaints. The leaf, flower and roots all make quite serviceable and effective teas, infusions and tinctures. Make sure to strain out the small hairs from the leaves before consumption. The leaves can also be prepared as an herbal smoke blend.

HERBAL SUBSTITUTES: Mugwort (*Artemisia vulgaris*): inhalation | horsetail (*Equisetem arvense*): connective tissue

SAFETY AND PRECAUTIONS

Mullein is generally considered safe. If you are pregnant, nursing or taking prescription medication, please consult your physician before taking this or any other herb.

LOOK-ALIKES: Lamb's ear (*Stachys byzantina*), foxglove (*Digitalis purpurea*) TOXIC

IDENTIFY & GROW

🌸 **TYPE OF PLANT**: Biennial

🌸 **HABITAT**: Mullein likes bright sunny places, and it can thrive in a variety of soil conditions due to a substantial tap root.

🌸 **HEIGHT**: 2–8' (0.6–2.5 m)

🌸 **LEAF**: During mullein's first year of growth, it forms a basal rosette of fuzzy, gray-green leaves. During its second year, a tall spike emerges with leaves alternating up the stem, becoming smaller near the flowers.

🌸 **STEM**: Tall, erect stem with leaves "clutching" and funneling water to the roots of the plant

🌸 **FLOWER**: Tall, terminal flower spikes with many five-petaled yellow flowers. Flowers start blooming at the base of the spike near mid-summer and travel toward the top as the season progresses.

🌸 **GROWING INFORMATION**: Mullein seeds can be sown in early spring into well-mulched soil in a sunny spot and kept lightly moist until well established.

🌸 **FORAGE OR GROW?** While I may consider mullein an attractive, even stately plant, others may not regard it so well. I think that this is an herb to forage, although it is very important to harvest from a contaminant-free area as mullein is a bio-accumulator of heavy metals from the earth. Avoid harvesting from industrial sites, roadsides and heavily logged areas.

BEST HARVEST PRACTICES

FLOWER HARVEST WINDOW: Summer

LEAF HARVEST WINDOW: Summer

ROOT HARVEST WINDOW: Early fall

Leaves should be gathered at the basal rosette stage or early in the growing season of the second year. Roots are ideally harvested during fall of the first year. Flowers should be collected in intervals throughout the blooming season.

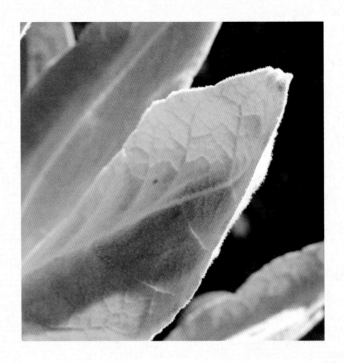

TIP: Mullein is often found at abandoned industrial sites. As this botanical is a bio-accumulator of heavy metals, it is best to avoid harvest from possibly contaminated areas.

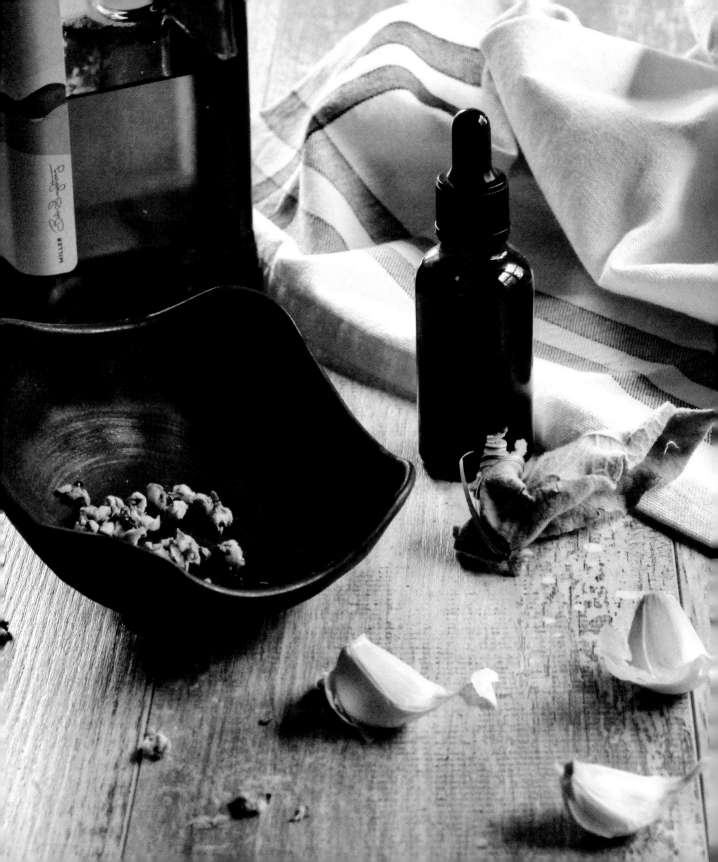

MULLEIN FLOWER OIL FOR ACHY EARS

Mullein flowers are an excellent way to give speedy pain relief to achy ears. Not only will this oil relieve pain from a minor ear infection, it will also help to decrease the pressure in one's ears due to sinus and lymph congestion. Garlic may also be added to increase its infection-fighting abilities.

This recipe is safe for adults and children.

YIELD: 4 ounces (120 ml)

INGREDIENTS

½ cup (120 ml) olive oil

1 tbsp (1 g) dried mullein flowers

1 tsp dried garlic granules (optional)

INSTRUCTIONS

Combine the ingredients and use one of the infusion methods listed on page 12. When the infusion is complete, strain through two layers of flower sack cloth into a liquid measuring cup. Pour into 1- or 2-ounce (30- or 60-ml) amber glass dropper bottles. Use within 1 year.

To use: Place 1 to 3 drops in the ear canal. Do not use if the ear drum is perforated by a previous injury or infection.

MULLEIN RESPIRATORY SMOKE

Respiratory smoke. It would seem an oxymoron, but it is actually an excellent way of delivering soothing benefits directly where they are needed—in the lungs and bronchial area. For smokers, try a blend of mullein and catmint as a tobacco replacement to soothe tension and suppress nicotine fits. For those dealing with mild respiratory irritations, sore throats and unproductive coughs, try the sage and mullein combination.

For best results, use freshly dried mullein that is light, soft and fluffy. Avoid crunchy, browned and overly dried mullein leaves.

YIELD: varies

INGREDIENTS

4 parts dried mullein leaf

1 part dried catmint or sage

INSTRUCTIONS

Blend the herbs together, and store in a tight-lidded jar. Use immediately.

To use: To smoke, pack the blend into a pipe, roll into cigarettes or simply burn a small amount of the blend in a small dish while standing over the dish and inhaling deeply.

This remedy is best suited for adults, and it should be limited to no more than 3 times daily.

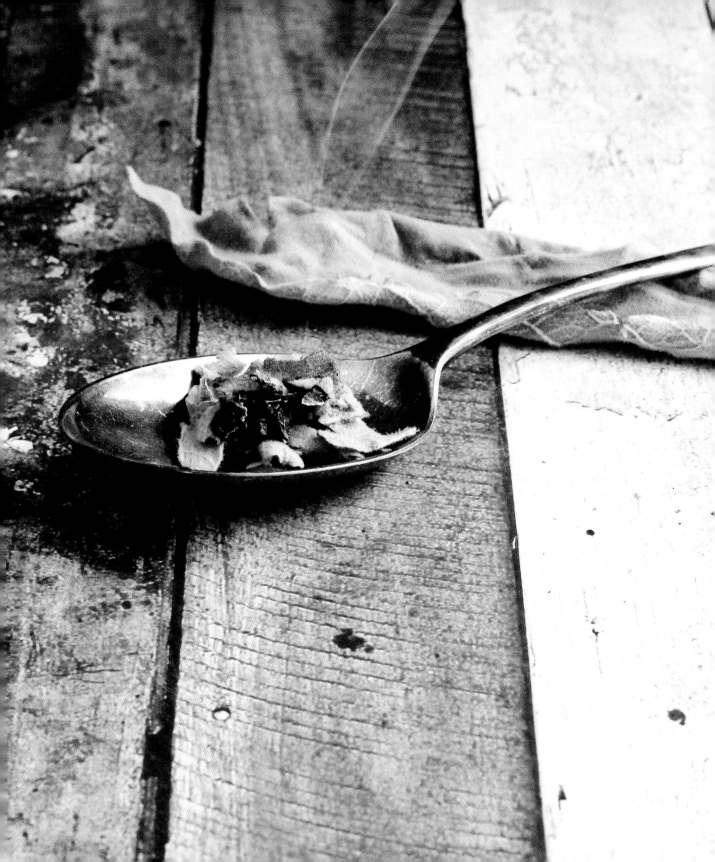

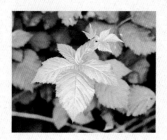

BLACKBERRY

OTHER COMMON NAMES: bramble, marionberry, lingonberry, boysenberry

LATIN NAME: *Rubus* sp.

HERBAL ENERGETICS: cool/dry

THERAPEUTIC ACTIONS: anti-inflammatory, antimicrobial, antioxidant, antispasmodic, astringent, diaphoretic, hypoglycemic, nutritive, styptic, tonic

PARTS USED: leaf, root, berries (edible)

HERBAL MONOGRAPH

It should come as no surprise that this botanical lands safely in the "nutritive" comfort zone. Blackberry leaves and roots contain a host of phytonutrients, as well as vitamins C and K and the minerals iron and manganese. As such I find blackberry preparations to be very effective for those in recovery-type conditions, such as dealing with the aftereffect of diarrhea and food poisoning, or those needing to restore iron levels due to blood loss and anemia. The berries are also considered highly nutritive and contain heart-friendly anthocyanins.

Old texts often point to the use of blackberry leaves and root for oral concerns. Blackberry was used to address concerns of spongy inflamed gums, bleeding gums and mouth sores and ulcerations. It is very soothing for sore throats, especially those for whom coughing and swallowing feel like shards of glass are dragging through one's airways.

Blackberry is uniquely well suited to complaints of the digestive system. Its astringent qualities help to arrest the loss of fluids through the intestinal wall during bouts of diarrhea. Additionally, blackberry is indicated for hemorrhoids, irritable bowel (with diarrhea), colitis and Crohn's disease. A recent study even suggests that blackberry leaf extract can decrease the bacterial counts of *H. pylori*, a bacterium associated with stomach cancer.

Due to its high presence of tannins and its antioxidant properties, a cooled decoction or infusion of blackberry leaf is extremely soothing to severe sunburns, especially those that are weepy and blistered. Blackberry is also suggested to smooth scaly skin conditions, such as eczema and psoriasis. With slight styptic qualities, this botanical is also excellent for slow bleeding, oozy wounds and blisters.

BEST PREPARATIONS: Blackberry leaf is ideally suited to herbal infusions and teas, while the roots deserve a decoction to extract their therapeutic benefits. Tinctures of low alcohol content and oxymels are also effective for the extraction of the nutritive and medicinal constituents.

HERBAL SUBSTITUTES: Raspberry (*Rubus idaeus*)

SAFETY AND PRECAUTIONS

Due to its high tannin content, limit use to no more than 3 cups (710 ml) of tea a day for no longer than a week of continual use. Allow for a one-week break before resuming.

LOOK-ALIKES: Raspberry (*Rubus idaeus*)

IDENTIFY & GROW

TYPE OF PLANT: Perennial

HABITAT: Highly adaptive, blackberry will thrive in a variety of conditions, including full sun to the moderate shade of an open forest. This botanical will naturalize in areas of poor soil.

HEIGHT: Trailing habit with vines reaching lengths of 20'+ (6 m)

LEAF: Dark green leaves; new, emerging growth may be red-bronze; palmate with 5 to 7 lobes and serrated margins

STEM: Prickly stems, trailing

FLOWER: White to pink five-petaled flowers bloom late spring through early summer

FRUIT: Fruit turns from green to black-purple as it ripens; juicy. Retain pithy white center when picked.

GROWING INFORMATION: Blackberries can be divided and planted in spring or fall. Leaves emerge on primocanes during the first year, and fruit on the matured floracanes the following year.

FORAGE OR GROW? Wild blackberry is available in many temperate regions, making it perfect for foraging. If growing in the home garden, take special care to prevent it from overtaking your garden.

BEST HARVEST PRACTICES

HARVEST WINDOW: Leaves can be harvested throughout the growing season. Berries should be picked when sweet and ripe, pulling easily away from stem. Roots can be dug, cleaned and sliced for drying in early fall.

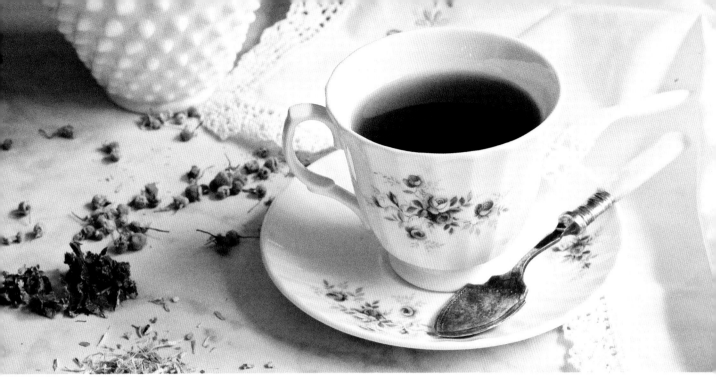

CALM YOUR BOWELS BLACKBERRY   & CHAMOMILE INFUSION

We've all been there. Whether from tainted takeout or the nefarious norovirus, we have all been hit with a case of the big D at some point in our lives. That's DIARRHEA, if you aren't familiar with my vernacular.

So, when your guts are in turmoil and you're not venturing too far from the bathroom, you need an herbal remedy to act fast to, ahem, slow things down a little. A decoction of blackberry root, then infused with blackberry leaves and chamomile will help to soothe and restore tone and balance to beleaguered bowels.

YIELD: 1 serving

INGREDIENTS

3 cups (710 ml) water

1 tbsp (3 g) dried blackberry root

1½ tsp (1 g) dried blackberry leaf

1½ tsp (1 g) dried chamomile

INSTRUCTIONS

Place the water and blackberry root in a small saucepan. Bring to a simmer. Simmer until the liquid has been reduced by approximately half of its original volume, about 10 to 15 minutes. When adequately reduced, remove from the heat. Add the blackberry leaf and chamomile to the decoction. Infuse for a minimum of 20 minutes, then strain and serve. Use immediately.

This preparation is safe for adults and children. Drink one serving up to 3 times daily.

DANDELION

OTHER COMMON NAMES: dent de lion, lion's tooth, milk witch, piss-en-lit, puffball

LATIN NAME: *Taraxacum officinale*

HERBAL ENERGETICS: cool/dry

THERAPEUTIC ACTIONS: alterative, anodyne (flower), antiarthritic, anti-inflammatory, aperitif, cholagogue, digestive, diuretic, emollient (flower), hepatic, laxative (root-mild), lithotryptic, nutritive, tonic

PARTS USED: all parts

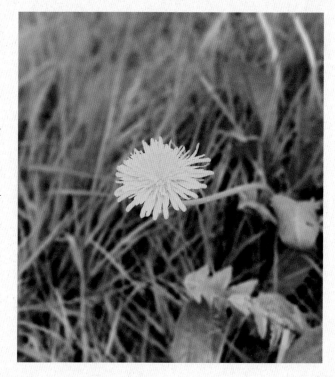

HERBAL MONOGRAPH

Never has a plant met the grisly blades of a lawn mower only to rise, rise, rise again like the dandelion. Dandelion is an optimistic herb with a sunny disposition. It is the reliable friend with a big smile, a warm heart and determined spirit. I am sure that even the most ardent landscapers would admit that blowing the dandelion summer seed fluff from the stems is necessary nurturing of one's inner child!

Ever generous, this much-maligned yard pest is one of the herbalist's best allies. From bright yellow blooms, to glorious green leaves, to the end of its long tap roots, dandelions are medicinal from head to toe.

To extol the many virtues of the embattled dandelion, one must start somewhere, and that somewhere shall be the roots. Dandelion roots are the storehouse of a multitude of therapeutic actions that influence one's health and well-being. In an age when we are growing increasingly aware of the importance of gut health, dandelion roots provide a very important prebiotic starch known as inulin. Inulin acts as an energy source for beneficial gut microbes. A properly nourished gut biome contributes to a variety of outcomes such as proper digestion, nutrient absorption and even good mental health. Additionally, the consumption of 10 grams of inulin a day appears to contribute to a significant reduction in blood lipids and regulation of blood glucose, according to a 2000 study.

Dandelion is revered as an herb for the liver within all the holistic modalities. It is particularly useful when there are signs of a hot, inflamed liver with stagnation. These signs may include:

- abdominal bloating
- increased visceral fat
- halitosis
- coated tongue
- mood swings with a tendency toward anger
- chemical sensitivity
- difficulty digesting fats

- cravings
- night sweats
- insomnia
- irregular bowel movements
- cravings
- PMW/estrogen dominance
- skin complaints (itchy red skin, rosacea, acne)
- fluid retention, gall stones
- headache, dry mouth
- bloodshot eyes
- yellowing skin

Dandelion appears to improve liver function and aid the natural detoxification process, while also protecting liver cells from oxidation and damage. A 2015 study of lab rats with induced acetaminophen toxicity demonstrated that those rats receiving an ethanol extract of dandelion root had a measurable reduction in liver damage compared to the control group.

Moving up the plant, we come to the lovely green leaf. When I think about dandelion leaf, my focus turns to all matters of good digestion. Dandelion leaves have a clear affinity for the gallbladder and, as such, aid in the digestion of fats. The greens stimulate the flow of gastric juices and increase the excretion of bile. Dandelion is ideal for those with "sour stomachs," a tendency toward belching and appetites often suppressed by the dread of indigestion. Dandelion leaf is also a strong diuretic, helping to drain the kidneys and bladder of retained fluids.

Dandelion leaves are also incredibly nutritious. They are an excellent source of vitamin A, while also offering vitamins C and B$_6$, as well as magnesium, calcium, iron, phosphorus, potassium and folate. With such a diverse nutrient profile, dandelion is an excellent tonic herb that supports and promotes all-around good health and vigor.

Dandelion's medicinal use does not stop with the leaf and the root. Their sunny yellow, characteristic flowers are often considered a tonic for the eyes, largely owing to their lutein and beta-carotene. As an emollient, moisturizing and pain-relieving herb, dandelion flowers make for the most appropriate salve for sore and chapped garden-weary hands with comfrey (see page 33). Even the sap that bleeds from a split stem is thought to help warts disappear and reduce the scarring and severity of acne.

BEST PREPARATIONS: Dandelion is such a versatile herb with a variety of potential medicinal preparations. Roots can be tinctured, either fresh or dried, and teas and infusions can be prepared from the dried root. Roasted dandelion root can serve as an herbal alternative to your daily cup of coffee. Leaves are ideally tinctured while fresh, and teas can be prepared with dried leaves. After wilting or drying individual flower petals, the slender yellow rays can be infused in a base oil for the creation of nourishing salves and creams. The milky sap can be applied directly to skin.

Tender young leaves make a tasty salad green; take care to harvest while still young, as older leaves may become bitter and unpalatable. Dandelion flowers are also edible, sometimes dipped in a batter and fried for a crispy fritter, or the petals tossed into cookie dough and pastries. Dandelion blossom wine is an old-fashioned favorite for wildflower wine and mead makers alike. Unopened blooms can be picked and pickled for a caper-like treat.

HERBAL SUBSTITUTES: Burdock (*Arctium lappa*) | yellow or curly dock (*Rumex* spp.)

SAFETY AND PRECAUTIONS
Dandelion should be avoided by those who are pregnant and nursing or those suffering from gallstones. Those with allergies to plants in the *Asteraceae* (daisy) family should not use dandelion, and latex allergy sufferers should avoid contact with its sap.

LOOK-ALIKES: Cat's ear (*Hypochaeris radicata*), false dandelion (*Agoseris glauca*), sow thistle (*Sonchus arvensis*), mouse ear hawkweed (*Hieracium pilosella*)

IDENTIFY & GROW

TYPE OF PLANT: Perennial

HABITAT: Dandelions are often in the lawn and in rich, relatively well-drained beds. They tend to grow in full sun to part shade and prefer slightly moist, but not wet or boggy soils.

HEIGHT: 8–12" (20–30 cm)

LEAF: Hairless, deeply serrated, pinnate leaves forming a basal rosette

STEM: Hollow stem with milky sap

FLOWER: Roughly 200 slender golden ray florets arrange as a composite appearing spring through early fall

SEED: Spherical plumes following flower

GROWING INFORMATION: Dandelion seeds should be sown in deep soil in early spring and kept slightly moist until germination. Once established, dandelions will reliably reappear year after year as long as some root segment is left in the soils after harvest.

FORAGE OR GROW? Why of course you should grow your own dandelions—so long as your neighbors are on board with your herbal endeavors. All jokes aside, this herb does equally well in a cultivated or wild setting. Advantages of growing ensure that you harvest from a contamination-free zone; disadvantages include cranky neighbors, spouses and homeowner associations.

BEST HARVEST PRACTICES
FLOWER AND LEAF HARVEST WINDOW: Spring and early summer

ROOT HARVEST WINDOW: Early fall

Early leaf growth should be harvested while still young to reduce bitterness. Flowers can be harvested after the morning dew has dried on sunny days. Roots are best carefully lifted with a small spade in the early fall, then scrubbed, rinsed, chopped and dried for future use.

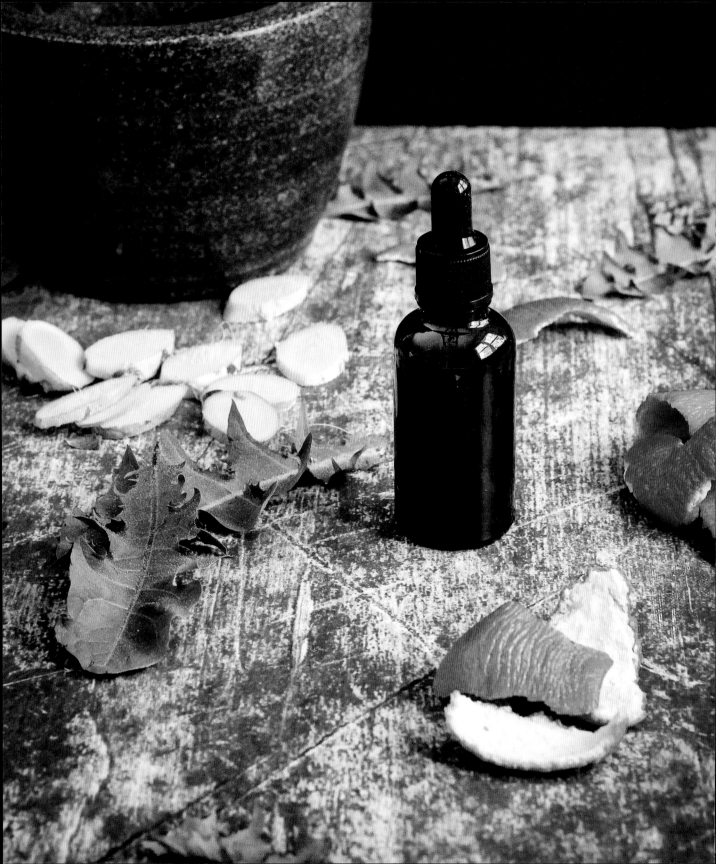

DIGESTIVE BITTERS WITH DANDELION, ORANGE PEEL & GINGER

Digestive discomforts can be mild to unbearable. From overeating and mild indigestion to heartburn and acid reflux, sufferers of frequent digestive upset need a bitters blend that hits all the marks. And one that tastes good to ensure compliance!

Enter dandelion greens to promote the flow of digestive juices, orange peel whose high pectin content discourages overeating and ginger to stimulate the peristalsis action of the stomach wall. These three herbs are a surefire way to get your digestion on the right track when taken before a meal. These digestive bitters can be taken straight, added into a small glass of water or even added to a cocktail or club soda.

YIELD: 1 pint (480 ml)

ADULT DOSE: 1–3 droppers full (1.5–4.5 ml), taken before meals

CHILD'S DOSE, AGES 6–12: ½–1 dropper full (0.75–1.5 ml), taken before meals

NOT RECOMMENDED FOR CHILDREN UNDER THE AGE OF 6.

INGREDIENTS

2 cups (480 ml) 100 proof spirits (vodka recommended)

¾ cup (40 g) chopped fresh dandelion greens

1 tbsp (6 g) finely chopped fresh ginger

Rind of 1 small orange (with pith)

INSTRUCTIONS

In a small blender, combine the spirits, dandelion greens, ginger and orange rind. Blend until it becomes a well-combined slurry. Transfer to a jar with a tight-fitting lid, and infuse for a minimum of 6 weeks.

After the infusion is complete, strain through two layers of flour sack cloth into a liquid measuring cup. Bitters may be slightly thick due to the presence of pectin; this is normal—just allow extra time for it to filter through the cloth. Pour into 1- or 2-ounce (30- or 60-ml) amber glass dropper bottles or into a pint-sized (480-ml) amber glass master bottle for dispensing. Use within 1 year.

DANDELION ROOT HERBAL COFFEE WITH BURDOCK, CHICORY & SPICES

Many of us live in a state of over-caffeination and stress. While there are benefits to coffee, the downsides are profound too. Too much coffee and you are shaky and "wired"—too little and you are sluggish with an unbearable headache. Even if some of us can kick the caffeine addiction, we still miss the "ritual" of coffee. Yeah, I like to make coffee and have the smell of freshly brewed coffee waft through my home. Don't you?

This herbal coffee blend offers the dark roasted flavors that I love in my favorite beans, but without the jitters and afternoon coffee headaches! A low, slow roasting in the oven develops deep, dark flavor in the roots, and the addition of cacao nibs and cinnamon chips adds even more depth of flavor remarkably reminiscent of actual coffee! For those needing to wean themselves from regular java, a blend of half coffee grounds and half herbal coffee blend is perfectly lovely! Best of all, the completed herbal blend can be prepared just as you would a regular ole pot of morning joe!

YIELD: approximately 1 pound (454 g)

INGREDIENTS

5 oz (142 g) dried dandelion root

5 oz (142 g) dried chicory root

3 oz (85 g) dried burdock root

1½ oz (43 g) cacao nibs

1½ oz (43 g) cinnamon chips

INSTRUCTIONS

Preheat the oven to 275°F (135°C, or gas mark 1).

Spread the dandelion, chicory and burdock roots out onto a rimmed baking sheet. Roast in the oven for approximately 2 hours, stirring about every 15 to 20 minutes. Roots are adequately roasted when they are somewhat brown and have a toasty fragrance. Remove from the oven, and set aside to cool.

In the bowl of a food processer or blender, add the cooled roasted roots, cacao nibs and cinnamon chips. Pulse until the mixture resembles the texture of coffee grounds, taking care not to produce too fine of a powder. Transfer your ground herbal coffee blend to a jar with a tight-fitting lid and prepare as you would a regular pot of coffee. Use more of the blend if you prefer dark roast, less if you lean toward lighter notes. Use within 6 months.

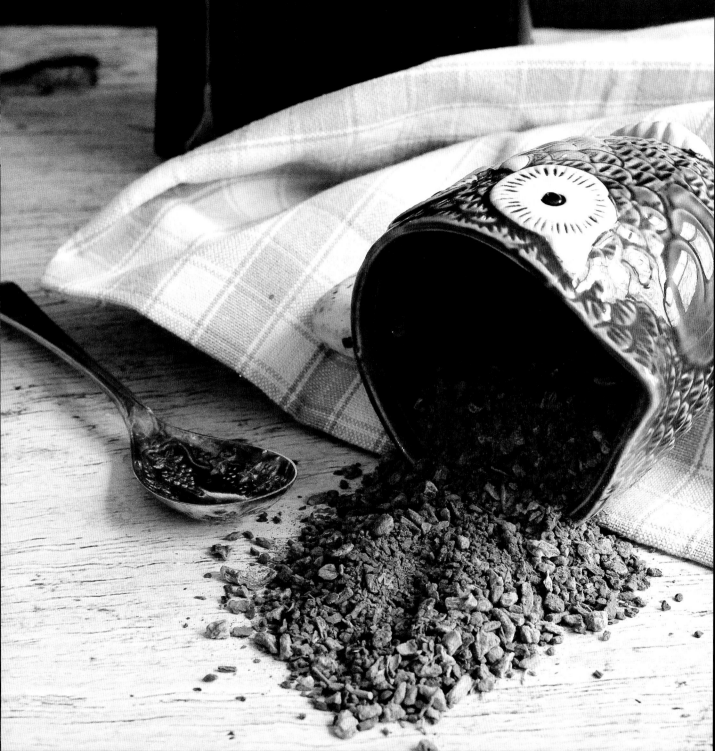

BURDOCK

OTHER COMMON NAMES: beggar's buttons, cocklebur, cockle buttons, thorny burr, gobo root

LATIN NAME: *Arctium lappa*

HERBAL ENERGETICS: cool/neutral

THERAPEUTIC ACTIONS: alterative, antibacterial, anti-inflammatory, anti-rheumatic, diaphoretic, diuretic, hepatic, hypoglycemic, laxative (mild), lymphatic, nutritive, prebiotic

PARTS USED: root, leaves, seeds

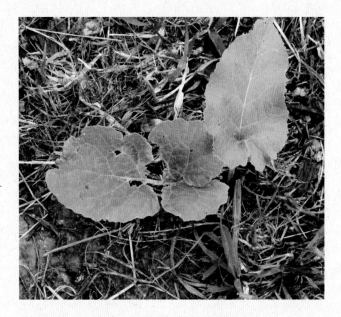

HERBAL MONOGRAPH

If you are a pet or livestock owner, you have undoubtedly come across burrs matted in the hair of your pet. Or in my case, matted the mane of your child's waist-length hair. It is practically impossible to not curse burdock while plucking the stubborn burrs off an irritable dog or a fussy toddler. But burrs are an occupational hazard that I will gladly deal with, for the medicinal benefits of burdock far outweigh the frustration of its well-defended seeds.

Burdock, simply said, is one of the most useful herbs in the apothecary for restoring health and wellness of the body and mind. It is an herb that demonstrates with incredible fortitude that herbs do not need to be exotic, rare or even beautiful to offer healing. Burdock teaches that the best medicine is the one that is available to you, right where you are.

Burdock is known in holistic circles as an "alterative" herb. Alterative is a concept that is difficult to sum up in a glossary-esque definition. They are herbs that alter the physical state. They are often associated with organs of elimination such as the kidneys, liver and bowels. Alterative herbs often have an affinity for the lymphatic system. Cleaning, clearing and moving are words that we often see used to describe the action of alterative herbs, burdock being chief among them. From Western Herbalism, to Traditional Chinese medicine and Ayurvedic modalities, burdock is upheld as an extraordinary herb for health.

Burdock's benefits are far reaching and apply to many organs and organ systems. It is an herb that supports the detoxification process. As such, it is an herb that acts on the liver. Burdock supports the liver's natural detoxification process. This herb is a valuable addition to formulas geared toward clearing a congested liver resulting from imbalanced hormones, poor eating habits, compromised organs of elimination, medication and drug and alcohol use/abuse. Liver congestion often reveals itself through externally observed symptoms such as red, rash-y splotches; acne (particularly deep, cystic acne); dry, scaly skin and imbalanced oil levels (excessively dry or excessively oily skin). Internally, liver congestion may manifest itself in excessive levels of certain hormones such as estrogen, high cholesterol levels, elevated uric acid and acidosis. Burdock assists the liver-supporting toxin elimination through the skin, bowel and urinary tract. Additionally, herbalists have long used burdock to address hepatitis concerns, and recent studies have shown that isolated burdock constituents have an inhibitory effect on the virus.

Beyond burdock's action on the liver, this botanical offers benefits for the digestive system that are somewhat unique. It acts on the gallbladder to stimulate bile production, making it an excellent herb for those who have difficulty digesting fats. It is also helpful for those who are plagued by constipation with hard, dry stools. Burdock root contains an insoluble starch called inulin that serves two very important functions for the digestive system, and by default, the whole body. Inulin is an excellent prebiotic for the beneficial microbes in the gut. A prebiotic is a substance that provides food and fuel to the microbes so that they can carry out their essential function. Secondly, inulin, as its name may suggest, helps to stabilize blood glucose levels, making burdock a vital herb for those who experience spikes and crashes following carbohydrate-heavy meals. As such, burdock has been linked to many long-term health benefits, such as decreased inflammation and cancer risk (which are associated with excessive blood glucose levels).

Burdock is often suggested as an herb to remedy a variety of skin complaints, from dry skin to sebaceous cysts. Although the mechanism by which burdock benefits the skin is somewhat unclear, there are a couple of schools of thought that have strong merit. It is believed that skin complaints are manifestations of poor liver health, so in supporting liver function, skin complaints naturally resolve. Additionally, many herbalists are inclined to believe that burdock helps to regulate sebum—the oily, lubricating substances secreted in the skin—production, by down-regulating excessive sebum and increasing insufficient supply.

BEST PREPARATIONS: All burdock parts can be prepared a variety of ways. The root is best decocted or tinctured, while the leaf and seeds can be prepared as a tea, infusion or tincture. Oil infusion can also be prepared using dried plant matter.

Burdock root is an excellent root vegetable and can be prepared like a carrot or parsnip. I also like to roast the dried root to prepare an herbal coffee substitute (see page 76).

HERBAL SUBSTITUTES: Dandelion root (*Taraxacum officinale*): hepatic

SAFETY AND PRECAUTIONS
Burdock may speed up the metabolism of certain medication such as contraceptives, antidepressants and statins. If you are pregnant, nursing or taking prescription medication, please consult your physician before using this or any other herb.

LOOK-ALIKES: Dock (*Rumex* sp.)

IDENTIFY & GROW
   ❀ **TYPE OF PLANT:** Biennial

   ❀ **HABITAT:** Burdock tolerates full sun to partial shade and prefers deep rich soil with adequate moisture.

   ❀ **HEIGHT:** 2–6' (0.6–2 m)

   ❀ **LEAF:** Large arrow- or heart-shaped leaves with uneven, wavy margins, sometimes measuring over 2 feet (60 cm). Pink to light purple central ribs. Forms basal rosette during the first year.

   ❀ **FLOWER:** Second year plants produce small 1–2" (2.5–5-cm) spiny, thistle-like flowers

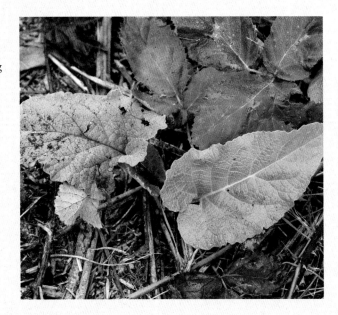

   ❀ **SEED:** Covered in spines; appears late summer through early fall

   ❀ **GROWING INFORMATION:** Burdock seeds are hardy and adaptive, and they can be sown directly as soon as the soil can be worked in the spring. Thin seedlings to one plant every 2 feet (60 cm) to prevent crowding.

   ❀ **FORAGE OR GROW?** Burdock is easily identified and grows prolifically. This is an herb to forage.

BEST HARVEST PRACTICES
LEAF HARVEST WINDOW: Spring and early summer

ROOT HARVEST WINDOW: Fall of first year's growth

Leaves can be gathered in either the first or second year throughout the growing season. Roots are ideally harvested from the first year's plant. Burrs can be gathered and dried in a paper bag, then pounded to separate the seed from the burr.

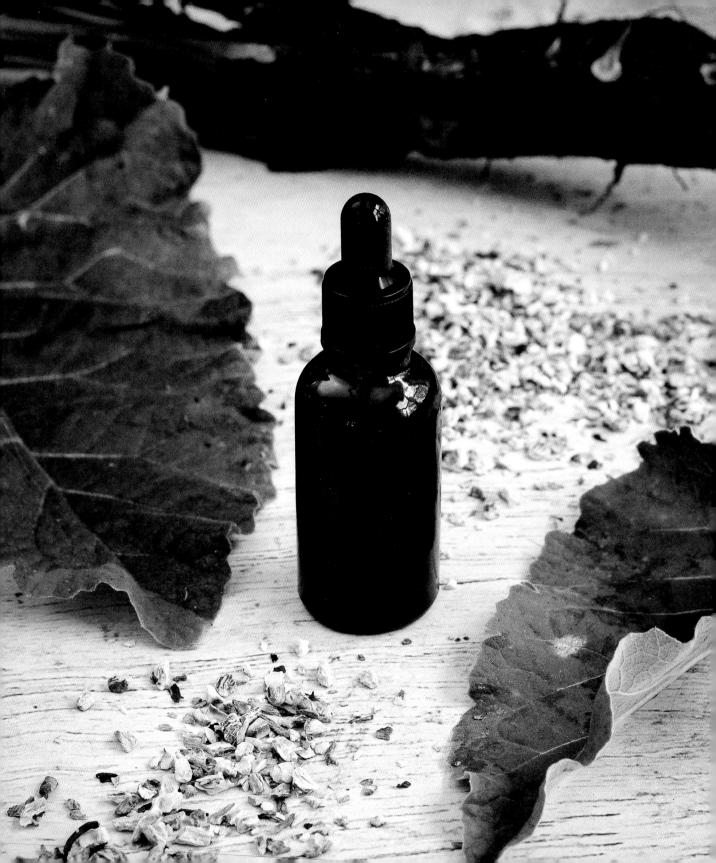

BURDOCK DETOXIFICATION TINCTURE

Burdock is a generous weed. Big broad leaves and a long taproot offer a substantial amount of medicine with every harvest. While burdock root often steals the scene with its noble liver-supporting action, I like to include burdock leaf in my detoxification tincture to harness some whole plant medicine. This tincture is ideal for those who show signs of a sluggish liver such as itchy, scaly skin, muddy complexion, acne and digestive issues.

YIELD: 1 pint (480 ml)

ADULT DOSE: 1–3 droppers full (1.5–4.5 ml), 3 times daily

CHILD'S DOSE: While burdock is safe for children, we generally do not see the need for hepatic herbs with young people. If your child is showing signs of liver damage or toxicity, please consult your physician.

INGREDIENTS

2 cups (480 ml) 100 proof spirits (vodka recommended)

½ cup (65 g) sliced fresh burdock root

½ cup (25 g) fresh burdock leaves, chopped finely

INSTRUCTIONS

Place the spirits, burdock root and leaves in a jar with a tight-fitting lid. Infuse the spirits with the burdock for a minimum of 6 weeks.

When the infusion is complete, strain through two layers of flour sack cloth into a liquid measuring cup. Pour into 1- or 2-ounce (30- or 60-ml) amber glass dropper bottles or a pint-sized (480-ml) amber glass master bottle for dispensing. Use within 1 year.

CHICKWEED

OTHER COMMON NAMES: chickwort, winterweed, starwort, adder's mouth

LATIN NAME: *Stellaria media*

HERBAL ENERGETICS: cool/moist

THERAPEUTIC ACTIONS: alterative, anti-obtrusant, anti-proliferative, anti-rheumatic, antiviral, demulcent, diuretic, expectorant, febrifuge (when person feels hot and agitated; not chilled), galactagogue, laxative (mild), vulnerary

PARTS USED: leaves, flower

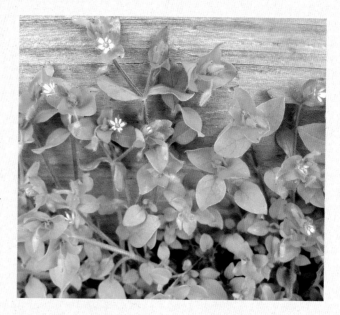

HERBAL MONOGRAPH

There are very few herbs that we can rely on to be abundant during late winter and early spring. Cold temperatures and wet conditions keep many intrepid foragers and their plant allies decidedly dormant during the gloom and doldrums. Yet there is one herb in particular worthy of donning the rain slicker and rubber boots for.

And her name is *Stellaria media*. Or you can call her chickweed.

It is perhaps not coincidental that chickweed arrives just about the time that we start feeling the need to spring clean—literally and figuratively. Although the air may be chill, I am always inclined to throw open a window or two on the rare dry day, and no more so than when I am purging the detritus of winter. Chickweed is a mover and a cleaner, of sorts. It is the botanical embodiment of spring cleaning. It is open windows and uncluttered surfaces. Just when the weight of the winter junk is making us feel heavy and sluggish, chickweed is raising her star-like countenance to the sky!

Chickweed has a deep affinity for the kidneys and the urinary tract. Although diuretic in nature, chickweed is particularly gentle and nondrying when used in moderation. Chickweed is an ideal herb for complaints of fullness about the pelvic region, retained water, irritable or weak bladder (especially postpartum or post-surgical), bladder infections and interstitial cystitis. It draws out heat, soothing inflamed tissues. Due to its saponin content (a soapy constituent that serves to increase absorption in stagnant and cystic tissues), chickweed is suggested as a remedy for benign ovarian cysts. Beyond that, chickweed has traditionally been associated with assisting one in losing weight and shrinking fatty deposits.

Chickweed is a nutritive green with an abundance of vitamins and minerals, making it a perfect tonic for restarting our systems. Vitamins A and C are in great supply with this botanical, as are a host of B vitamins, as well as minerals such as calcium, magnesium and zinc. The high chlorophyll content helps restore oxygen to the blood, helping one to feel more vibrant and refreshed.

Another, perhaps often overlooked, use for chickweed is that of expectorant. Not only does it work to soothe a dry, hot, spasmodic cough, but chickweed will also aid in the expectoration of mucus lodged in lung tissue. This little plant is ideal for those with a lingering, irritating and unproductive cough.

Another virtue of chickweed is its ability to draw out heat, swelling and infection. External application for boils, blisters, splinters and even swollen lymph glands will aid in the removal of irritants while cooling inflamed and painful tissues. Poultices applied to ulcerations can help with the severity of fever blisters and herpes simplex virus sores.

BEST PREPARATIONS: Chickweed lends itself to a variety of applications due to its complex profile of both water- and fat-soluble constituents. Its unassuming and vague flavor make it a serviceable tea or infusion with little objection—and it is even better when combined with more flavorful herbs such as lemon verbena or turned into a delicious, nutritive broth with something like miso. This is an herb that should be tinctured fresh for best results. Poultices produced from either fresh or dry plant matter are also very effective.

Chickweed is a tasty herb to use in a mixed green salad as it lacks the overwhelming bitterness of many spring greens while also having a fleshy, toothsome bite. I like to fold the fresh spring growth into chèvre with chives and spread it on toast rounds for a savory snack. It is a wonderful herb to use in place of spinach in green smoothies.

HERBAL SUBSTITUTES: Cornsilk (*Zea mays*): urinary health | plantain (*Plantago* sp.): anti-obtrusant

SAFETY AND PRECAUTIONS
Although largely considered gentle and safe, chickweed should be avoided by those with kidney disease. If you are pregnant, nursing or taking prescription medication, please consult your physician before taking this or any other herb.

LOOK-ALIKES: Scarlet pimpernel (*Anagallis arvensis*)

IDENTIFY & GROW
🌸 **TYPE OF PLANT:** Annual

🌸 **HABITAT:** Chickweed loves to appear in previously cultivated soil and will thrive in the remains of last year's vegetable garden patch. It tolerates full sun during cool conditions or dappled shade; spring growth tends to die back when summer heat hits with potential for a fall flush of new growth in temperate regions.

🌸 **HEIGHT:** 3–7" (8–18 cm); sprawling

🌸 **LEAF:** Opposite, ovoid and fleshy, approximately ¼–1" (0.6–2.5 cm) in length

🌸 **STEM:** Long creeping, sapless stem with hairs running along one side of the stem, hairs alternating sides after each set of leaves. The core of the stem is an elastic, stretchy thread.

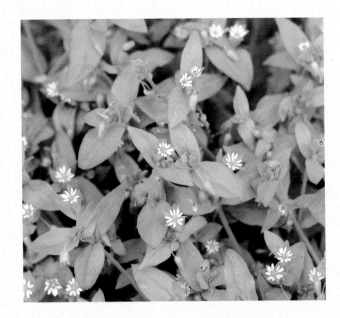

🌸 **FLOWER:** Five severely divided white petals that make it appear to have ten separate petals, in groups of three to five. Individual flowers have the appearance of a star.

🌸 **GROWING INFORMATION:** To cultivate, combine the tiny seeds with sand and broadcast over recently cultivated or raked soil in fall or early spring. Lightly top dress with topsoil or compost and keep moist until germination.

🌸 **FORAGE OR GROW?** Under the right conditions, such as an established garden plot, chickweed will likely volunteer itself, so this is an herb best to forage. However, if you want to establish a chickweed area that will reliably reseed, year after year, you can certainly grow this nutritious herb.

BEST HARVEST PRACTICES
LEAF HARVEST WINDOW: Late winter to early spring

Greens are most tender just before flowers start to open, at which point all the aerial parts are edible. For medicinal use, chickweed leaves can be gathered and removed from the stems before drying (discarding stems and any yellow or damaged leaves). Leaves can be blanched and frozen for future culinary uses.

SPRING CLEANING TONIC

Chickweed, combined with nettle and lemon verbena, makes for a lovely spring tonic in the vein of herbalist Susan Weed's "nourishing herbal infusions." This tonic is best prepared the night before and allowed to infuse overnight to extract all the nutritious and medicinal constituents. Strained and poured over ice with a slice or two of fresh lemon, this herbal infusion can be sipped throughout the day to make you feel lighter and brighter! Spring cleaning for the whole body!

YIELD: 4 cups (105 g) of dried herbs

ADULT DOSE: 16–32 oz (475–950 ml), daily

CHILD'S DOSE, AGES 6–12: 8–16 oz (240–475 ml), daily

NOT RECOMMENDED FOR CHILDREN UNDER THE AGE OF 6.

INGREDIENTS

2 cups (50 g) dried chickweed

1½ cups (35 g) dried nettle leaf

½ cup (20 g) dried lemon verbena

Lemon slices, for serving (optional)

INSTRUCTIONS

Mix the dried herbs together, and store in an airtight jar out of direct light.

To prepare the tonic, place 2 to 3 heaping tablespoons (3 to 5 g) of the herbal mixture into a 1-quart (1-L) jar. Pour water just off the boil to fill the jar. Allow the infusion to cool on the counter for 30 minutes before placing in the refrigerator overnight; this will avoid temperature stressing your jar.

In the morning, strain the infusion and pour over ice. If not consuming the entirety, any reserved infusion can be stored in the refrigerator for 24 hours. Add slices of lemon, if desired, and sip throughout the day. Use within 1 year.

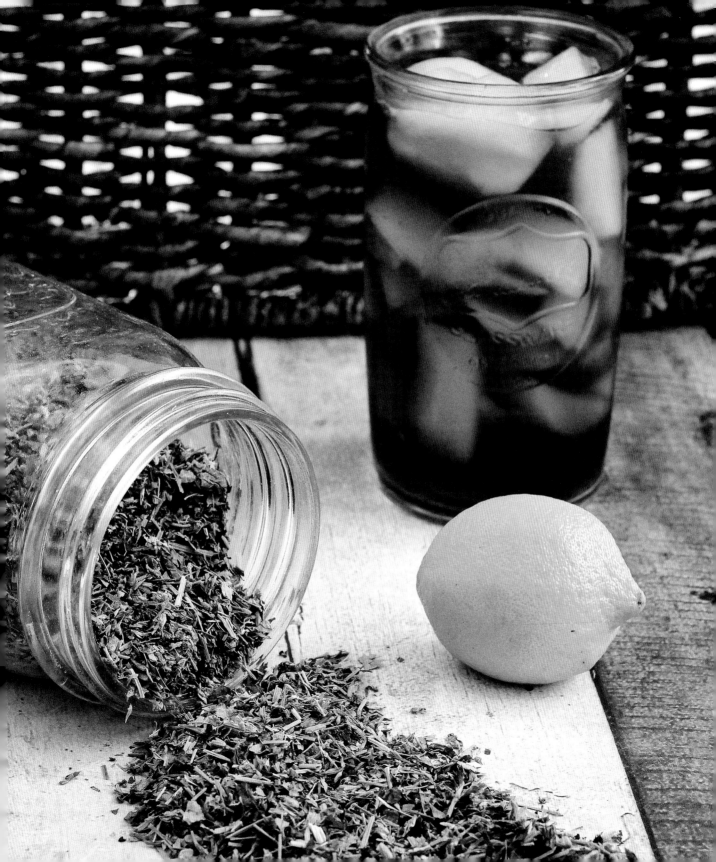

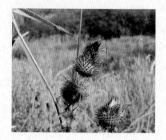

MILK THISTLE

OTHER COMMON NAMES: St. Mary's thistle, Marian thistle, holy thistle

LATIN NAME: *Silybum marianum*

HERBAL ENERGETICS: cool/neutral to moist

THERAPEUTIC ACTIONS: anti-inflammatory, antioxidant, cholagogue, demulcent, galactagogue, heptatoprotective, hepatic, tropho-restorative, immune-modulating

PARTS USED: seed, leaf (edible)

HERBAL MONOGRAPH

Thistle is often the bane of many gardeners, farmers and backwoods explorers. Tenacious and fearsome, the thorny leaves are the perfect defensive foil to its rather picturesque thistle. Some medicinal plants practically beg an intrepid herbalist to take them home, such as clingy cleavers. While others, such as milk thistle, take some careful finesse to coax into the home apothecary.

Milk thistle is known primarily for its strong affinity for the liver. Herbalists have long used milk thistle for complaints of the liver such as congestion (low catabolism), painful enlargement, alcoholism, hepatitis and cirrhosis. There is substantial European use of the intravenous silibinin (derived from milk thistle) for amanita mushroom poisoning, although it is not a remedy currently favored in most North American hospitals due to poor availability and lack of FDA approval. It should be noted that silibinin is a highly concentrated, standardized extract and that ingestion of milk thistle seeds and whole seed extracts are not an "at-home remedy" for amanita poisoning. Rather, I offer this information to demonstrate milk thistle's profound liver-protective potential.

Beyond the liver, milk thistle is considered an effective galactogogue—meaning that it may help to increase breast milk production. One particular study of 50 lactating women observed an approximately 50 percent increase in milk production with those receiving the extract silymarin compared to the placebo group. Furthermore, this was observed with no known side effects.

BEST PREPARATIONS: Milk thistle lends itself well to teas, infusions, encapsulations and tinctures. Milk thistle seeds can also be eaten when ground to a powder and incorporated into food and drink such as smoothies and granola.

HERBAL SUBSTITUTES: Dandelion root (*Taraxacum officinale*): hepatic | Fenugreek (*Trigonella foenum-graecum*): galactogogue

SAFETY AND PRECAUTIONS

Avoid using milk thistle if you take a medication that is metabolized by the liver. If you are pregnant, nursing or taking prescription medication, please consult your physician before taking this or any other herb.

LOOK-ALIKES: Bull thistle (*Cirsium vulgare*)

IDENTIFY & GROW

TYPE OF PLANT: Biennial

HABITAT: Milk thistle can be found in full sun, and it prefers rocky, dry soils that are slightly acidic.

HEIGHT: 2–6' (0.6–2 m)

LEAF: Leaves are oblong to lanceolate, either pinnate or lobate, with spiny margins.

STEM: Many branching stems with upper leaves cupping the stem

FLOWER: Purple thistle flowers that may be spiny, about 1–4" (2.5–10 cm) wide

SEED: Each flower produces approximately 200 brown seeds that are of relatively good size.

GROWING INFORMATION: As milk thistle is considered a noxious weed in many areas, you should contact your county extension office or municipality before planting. If planting, it is important to plant in a protected area to minimize its invasive nature, such as planting in a container protected from wind. Seeds can be sown directly in spring and will require frequent watering until established, after which they are somewhat drought resistant.

FORAGE OR GROW? Due to the aggressive nature of milk thistle, this is an herb to forage.

BEST HARVEST PRACTICES
SEED HARVEST WINDOW: Late summer to early fall

To gather seeds, harvest flowers as they start to dry on the plant but BEFORE they start to split open. Wearing gloves, carefully cut flowers from the stalk and place in a paper bag to dry for 7 to 10 days. When dried, crush each flower with a gloved hand to release the seeds. Note that the roots, leaf growth and flowers are all edible, but require a thorough de-spining in order to make them edible.

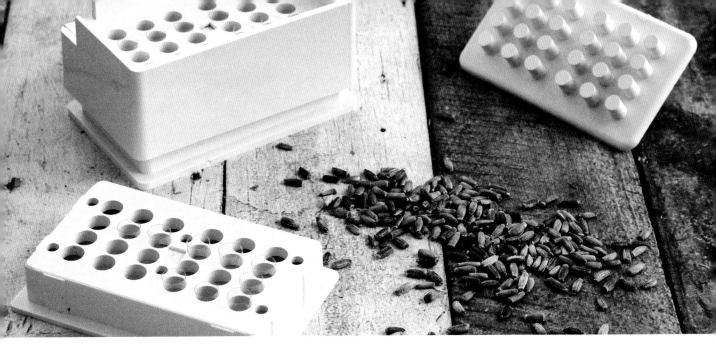

LIVER-PROTECTIVE MILK THISTLE CAPSULES

Truth be told, capsule making is one of my LEAST favorite herbal tasks. Even with my little capsule making tool, I find it to be a boring, repetitive task. It is the time to listen to a good podcast while attending to powdered herbs and small capsules. I reserve capsule making mainly for two reasons—for the most bitter and unpalatable of herbs and for those that are averse to or cannot tolerate alcohol. While tincturing is often my favored means of administration, it isn't always an appropriate choice. This is especially true for folks in recovery from alcohol and drug addiction. Milk thistle provides outstanding protective and restorative action on the liver, making it a wonderful herb for those looking to support their wellness after addiction.

YIELD: 120 capsules

ADULT DOSE: 2–3 capsules, 3 times daily

CHILD'S DOSE: While milk thistle is safe for children, we generally do not see the need for hepatic herbs with young people. If your child is showing signs of liver damage or toxicity, please consult your physician.

INGREDIENTS

1 ounce (28 g) milk thistle seeds

120 "00" capsules

INSTRUCTIONS

Using a dedicated coffee/spice grinder or a mortar and pestle, grind the milk thistle seeds to a fine powder. Using a capsule making tool or filling by hand, pack the milk thistle powder into the long end of the capsule and cap tightly. Store in an airtight container in a cool, dark place. Use within 1 year.

HAWTHORN

OTHER COMMON NAMES: May-tree, thornapple, whitethorn, hawberry

LATIN NAME: *Crataegus* sp.

HERBAL ENERGETICS: cool/dry

THERAPEUTIC ACTIONS: antiarrhythmic, antioxidant, antispasmodic, astringent, cardiovascular, carminative, diuretic, hypotensive, stimulant, vasodilator

PARTS USED: leaf, flower, berry, thorns (essence)

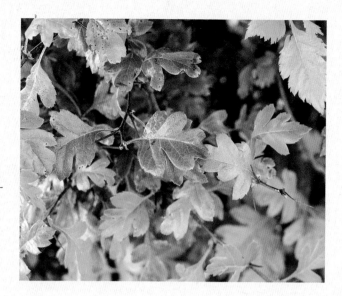

HERBAL MONOGRAPH

Perhaps rivaled only by rose, hawthorn is a much storied and fabled botanical. With many of its medicinal virtues supporting the physical heart, it should come as no great surprise that hawthorn lore is steeped in tales of the metaphorical heart as well. More specifically, hawthorn's allegory is deeply rooted in stories of protection. Protection of marriage unions, newborn babes and the family home. Legends speak to boundaries and thresholds, to the transition of seasons (particularly that of spring and fall), to fertility and to deep un-aging sleep. If we closely examine these more ephemeral, if whimsical, stories, we find a strong parallel to the medicinal virtue of the plant. Hawthorn is a botanical that "told" our ancestors what it was good for, long before science did.

Hawthorn is a plant that can teach us a lot about how to heal our bodies and minds by listening to nature, and to ourselves. One should see hawthorn for what it is—a sturdy and resolute tree or shrub, resistant to wind, growing in often harsh environments, offering its flowers and fruit only to those mindful enough to brave its thorns. Hawthorn teaches us about the importance of boundaries—we often see it planted in hedgerows and its noteworthy thorns forbid unwelcome visitors. Its lore teaches us about both literal and metaphorical thresholds, and it is associated with the Roman goddess of the doorway. Perhaps it is not a stretch to think of the heart as the great threshold of the body, through which passes our all-important blood.

It should come as no great surprise that a discussion of hawthorn would launch from its great medicinal benefits for the heart, and, more largely, the entire cardiovascular system. There are innumerable studies and countless anecdotal accounts demonstrating hawthorn's unique ability to support cardiovascular health. Hawthorn seems to help to regulate heartbeat and strengthen the muscle wall, making it an appropriate herb for concerns of arrhythmia, tachycardia and palpitations. It is particularly effective for hearts of red-faced, A-typed personalities, but is also a gentle support to those recovering from illness or addiction. It is also suggested for support in both congestive and non-congestive heart failure conditions.

One of hawthorn's most profound influences is on blood pressure. Herbalists find it to be the great equalizer. It is well known in both Western herbalism and traditional Chinese medicine for reducing elevated blood pressure, particularly that in which the diastolic reading is especially high. Older folk terms refer to hawthorn use for those with "high blood"— referring to people with flushed skin, meaty palms and a tendency toward perspiration, all indicating a saturated capillary bed. Hawthorn may also be an effective herbal remedy for those with a rapid pulse. This herb is even indicated for those suffering from insomnia, particularly those who can fall asleep but wake frequently, sometimes accompanied by a racing heart and night sweats.

We also find hawthorn to be a premiere herb for high cholesterol levels and undesirable lipid profiles. Both tradition and science suggest that hawthorn may be helpful in reducing low-density lipoprotein and high triglycerides, and may even help prevent arteriosclerosis by inhibiting oxidation and reducing inflammation. In strengthening the arterial wall, we also see hawthorn suggested for the prevention of varicose veins, as well as for increasing circulation for those with cold extremities.

BEST PREPARATIONS: Offering leaves, flowers, berries and even thorns, hawthorn is a botanical that lends itself to many preparations. The leaves, flowers and berries all make for a lovely tea and infusion. The berries can be used to craft a ruby-hued syrup. All mentioned parts make for an exceptional tincture, although I do like to note that as the berries have a high pectin content, I use a small amount of pectinase enzyme to reduce the viscosity that can sometimes be observed in hawthorn berry tinctures.

The berries can be creatively blended with other fruits for delicious jams and jellies, and hawthorn ketchup is a favorite of the wild foodie scene. The berries are often used for cordial making, and I have crafted a few beautiful bottles of rose hip and hawthorn mead in the past.

HERBAL SUBSTITUTES: Garlic (*Allium sativum*): lipid concerns | motherwort (*Leonurus cardiaca*): heart & circulation

SAFETY AND PRECAUTIONS
Hawthorn may potentiate other lipid-lowering and circulation-promoting medications. Please consult your physician before using hawthorn in conjunction with any heart- and cardiovascular related medications. If you are pregnant, nursing or taking prescription medication, please consult your physician before taking this or any other herb.

LOOK-ALIKES: Black haw (*Viburnum prunifolium*)

IDENTIFY & GROW
    TYPE OF PLANT: Deciduous tree or shrub

    HABITAT: A particularly adaptive botanical, hawthorn can be observed in a variety of soil conditions and prefers exposed, full-sun areas, although it is often seen at the edges of forested areas. It is a common hedgerow plant throughout Europe.

    HEIGHT: Full grown trees may reach 25–30' (7.5–9 m), although more shrubby varieties may be much shorter.

    LEAF: Spirally arranged 1–2" (2.5–5-cm) palmate, serrated green leaves with lighter underside; 3–5 lobes (deeply dissected about halfway to the midrib)

    FLOWER: Five-petaled white to slightly pink flowers emerge in May; sweet honey to slightly almond scent.

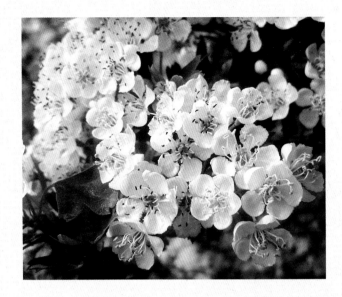

    FRUIT: Ovoid to round red fruits with a puckered blossom end. Thin skin surrounding a fleshy interior and three to five woody seeds. The fruit may be slightly blemished with darker spots.

    GROWING INFORMATION: Hawthorns make a lovely hedge or border as the shrubs and fully grown trees are quite stately. Trees can be planted from seeds, but to achieve sooner harvest it is best to plant seedling or hawthorn volunteers in an area with full sun, moderately loamy soils and enough water to establish a good root system.

    FORAGE OR GROW? I find hawthorn to be easy to find and identify, making it easy to forage, but it is a very pretty landscape plant that would not draw the ire of neighbors. Note: Hawthorn is not a tree-climbing plant for obvious reasons.

BEST HARVEST PRACTICES
FLOWER AND LEAF HARVEST WINDOW: Spring

BERRY HARVEST WINDOW: Fall

When harvesting flowers, keep in mind that you will be reducing the berry harvest come fall, so pick accordingly. Leaves and flowers should be gathered once the flowers begin to open, and berries are best harvested after the first frost. Superstitious types should note that it is considered unlucky to cut branches or bring them into the home. Some people gather thorns for energetic medicine from windfallen branches only.

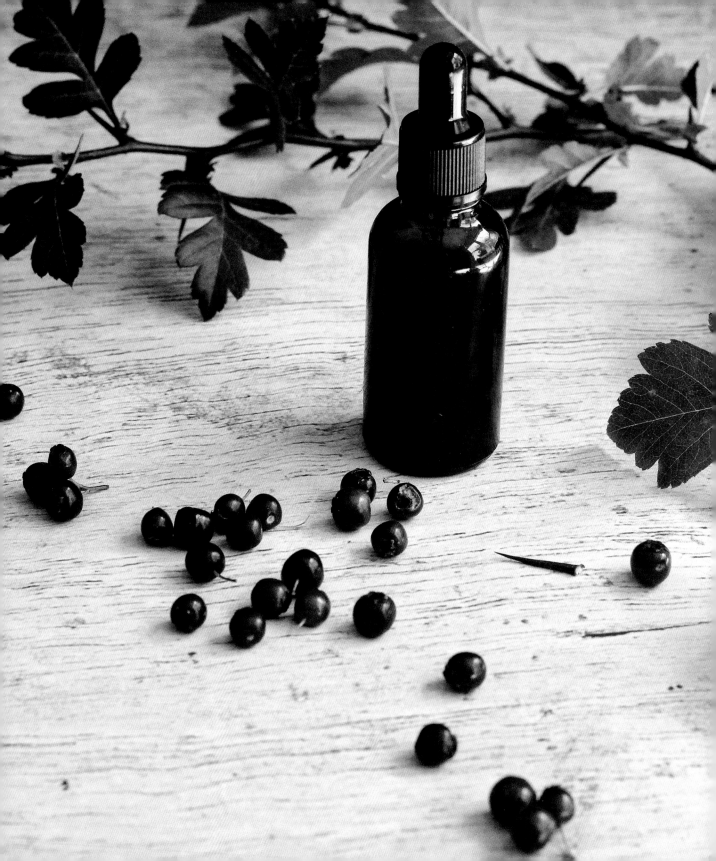

WHOLE HAWTHORN TINCTURE FOR CARDIOVASCULAR HEALTH

This is a two-part tincture that takes a little planning, a little patience and a little magic. This is a tincture for the physical heart, but it is also for the metaphorical heart. The combined actions of hawthorn flower, leaf and berry support cardiovascular health, while the inclusion of a single thorn is to help us manifest important boundaries. This is a tincture for both protection and healing. Leaves and flowers are gathered in spring, while berries and a thorn can be harvested in the fall. When both tinctures are adequately infused, they can be blended to create a very strong, yet gentle medicine.

YIELD: 1 quart (1 L)

ADULT DOSE: 1 dropper full (1.5 ml), 3 times daily

CHILDREN'S DOSE: While hawthorn is safe for children, we generally do not see the need for cardiovascular herbs with young people. If your child is showing signs of poor cardiovascular health or blood pressure issues, please consult your physician.

SPRING TINCTURE

2 cups (480 ml) 100 proof spirits (vodka recommended)

1½ cups (45 g) fresh hawthorn leaf and flower

FALL TINCTURE

2 cups (480 ml) 100 proof spirits (vodka recommended)

1½ cups (165 g) fresh hawthorn berries

1 hawthorn thorn, preferably from a windfallen branch

INSTRUCTIONS

During each season, infuse each tincture in jars with tight-fitting lids, shaking frequently, for a minimum of 6 weeks. When each tincture is complete, strain through two layers of flour sack cloth into a liquid measuring cup. The berry-thorn tincture may be somewhat viscous due to the presence of pectin in the berries.

Combine the spring and fall tinctures, and pour into a quart-sized (1-L) bottle for dispensing, or several 1- or 2-ounce (30- or 60-ml) amber glass dropper bottles. Use within 1 year.

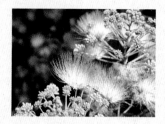

MIMOSA

OTHER COMMON NAMES: silk tree

LATIN NAME: *Albizia julibrissin*

HERBAL ENERGETICS: cool/dry

THERAPEUTIC ACTIONS: antidepressant, anxiolytic, hypotensive, sedative (mild)

PARTS USED: flower, bark

HERBAL MONOGRAPH

Few things make me as happy as a mimosa. Not the champagne cocktail—although there is an argument to be made for the sheer joy that bubbles offer—but rather the mimosa tree and its lovely blossoms. It is an exuberant tree, and it exudes happiness. I dare somebody not to smile when observing a mimosa in full flower. There is no question about its loveliness, unless you are living in an area where they are considered invasive, but more on that later. While most herbs that I cover have a multitude of therapeutic actions, mimosa has a refined focus. It focuses on restoring joy and protecting the heart, both emotional and physical.

Being that caring for the hurting and grief stricken takes a tender touch, I think we can all applaud Ms. Mimosa for being great at the most difficult thing. Not one to wear too many medicinal hats, mimosa has a sweet job to do, and it does it well.

Mimosa is a botanical that teaches us about the doctrine of signatures. Delicate, threadlike mimosa flowers appear from early to mid-summer and persist throughout much of the season. Due to their open, airy structure, mimosa blossoms are incredibly wind resistant despite their fragile appearance. Unlike a large, sturdy-looking blossom like a magnolia, stiff, damaging winds simply filter through mimosa blossoms instead of ripping the petals away. The tree persists in its joyful state, even in the face of trauma.

This botanical is often suggested for those reeling from grief and trauma. It is particularly sympathetic to those that feel locked up in their emotions and feel great difficulty in finding joy in life's pleasures. While it is very effective for helping people through traumatic experiences, such as the death of a loved one or a miscarriage, I find it to be a gentle herb to coax those who have grown calloused and indifferent, having never worked through pain.

On a more physiological side of matters, mimosa is a mild sedative and hypotensive. I find it to be calming to the wide-eyed panic one feels after an unexpected loss or trauma, quieting the racing heart and mind that struggles to find peace.

BEST PREPARATIONS: Flowers can be dried for tea or prepared as a tincture. Bark can also be used for tinctures and syrups.

HERBAL SUBSTITUTES: Hawthorn (*Crataegus* sp.): hypotensive

SAFETY AND PRECAUTIONS

Do not use mimosa if you are prone to manic episodes or are bipolar. If you are pregnant, nursing or taking prescription medication, please consult your physician before taking this or any other herb.

LOOK-ALIKES: Pasqueflower seedheads (*Pulsatilla* sp.)

IDENTIFY & GROW

TYPE OF PLANT: Deciduous tree

HABITAT: Mimosa trees grow best in sandy, somewhat alkaline soils in full sun. Wind resistant.

HEIGHT: Up to 40' (12 m)

LEAF: Green, fern-like, tripinnate leaves appear late spring

FLOWER: Pom-poms of fragrant, pink, threadlike stigmas appear mid-summer and persist for several weeks

SEED: Long, flat seed pods appear late summer through early fall

GROWING INFORMATION: Mimosa trees can be started from seed and can grow at a rate of approximately 3' (1 m) a year. They are very wind and cold resistant. They produce a lot of leaf and blossom litter, but are considered invasive in some areas. Short-lived tree—10 to 20 years.

FORAGE OR GROW? Mimosa can be foraged wild in many areas of eastern North America and from landscapes throughout temperate climates. If it does not grow wild and is legal to plant in your area, this is an easy plant to grow.

BEST HARVEST PRACTICES
FLOWER HARVEST WINDOW: Summer

Flowers can be collected throughout the blooming season before they start to wither. Bark can be scraped from branches.

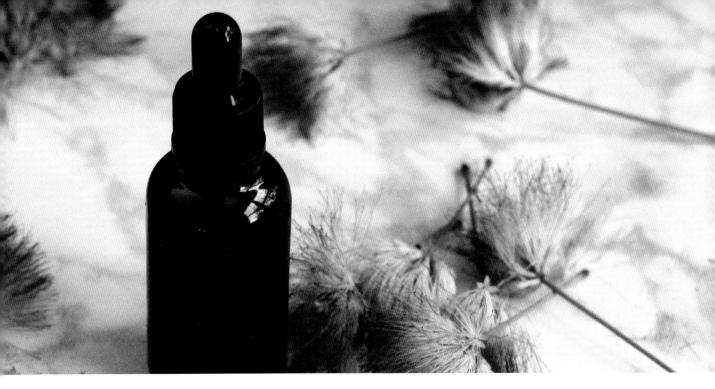

 ## MIMOSA ELIXIR FOR GRIEF & SADNESS

Mimosa is medicine for the eyes as well as a broken heart. It is a truly mesmerizing tree in full bloom, producing a generous froth of pinkish blooms. Harvesting mimosa blossoms is almost an act of healing in itself. Surrounded by delicate, fragrant blooms, it is hard not to find oneself uplifted by mimosa's beauty and generosity. Honey is added here because those who are suffering are deserving of small moments of sweetness.

YIELD: 1 pint (480 ml)

ADULT DOSE: 1–2 droppers full (1.5–3 ml), as needed

CHILD'S DOSE, AGES 6–12: 15–30 drops, as needed

CHILD'S DOSE, AGES 2–6: 5 drops, as needed

INGREDIENTS

2 cups (480 ml) 100 proof spirits (vodka recommended)

1½ cups (45 g) packed fresh mimosa blossoms

1 tbsp (15 ml) raw honey

INSTRUCTIONS

Combine the spirits and mimosa blossoms in a jar with a tight-fitting lid. Infuse for a minimum of 6 weeks, shaking daily. When the infusion is complete, strain through two layers of flour sack cloth into a liquid measuring cup. Add the honey, and stir vigorously to combine. Pour into 1- or 2-ounce (30- or 60-ml) amber glass dropper bottles or a pint-sized (480-ml) amber glass master bottle for dispensing. Use within 1 year.

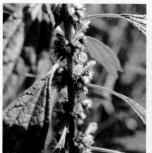
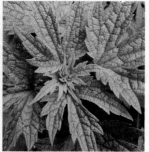

MOTHERWORT

OTHER COMMON NAMES: lion's tail, heart-wort

LATIN NAME: *Leonurus cardiaca*

HERBAL ENERGETICS: cool/dry

THERAPEUTIC ACTIONS: anti-inflammatory, antispasmodic, anxiolytic, astringent, cardiovascular, diaphoretic, digestive, diuretic, emmenagogue, hypotensive, nervine, stimulant, tonic, vermifuge

PARTS USED: aerial parts

HERBAL MONOGRAPH

Sometimes it is all in a name and never more so than with motherwort. As its common name would imply, motherwort is an herb with a profound affinity for female reproductive health. It is reached for when there are complaints of delayed and irregular menstruation. It may also help reduce and prevent menstrual cramping. It may also be a very helpful herb for young women who have anxiety and misplaced embarrassment about their menstrual periods. While motherwort is contraindicated for most of pregnancy, some traditional herbalists suggest its use in the final gestational weeks to tonify and strengthen the uterus for childbirth. Furthermore, it is a botanical tool of midwives to promote a strong labor, while also stimulating a lax, atonic uterus and aiding in the expulsion of a retained placenta following birth.

Motherwort is also an excellent remedy for concerns of hypertension and heart palpitations. It has long been considered a chief herb in formula throughout Western and Traditional Chinese Medicine for supporting good heart health and cardiovascular wellness. Motherwort is indicated when stress and anxiety contribute to heart palpitations and racing pulse.

Motherwort also acts on the digestive system and urinary tract. As a bitter, it stimulates the flow of digestive juices. It also helps to expel gastrointestinal parasites. Motherwort is also a gentle diuretic, aiding sluggish kidneys in urination. Perhaps most overlooked by modern practitioners is motherwort's effect on one's sense of self and well-being. This is an herb that I turn to when there are complaints of anxiety and panic attacks coupled with a lack of courage, meek temperament and suppressed "voice."

BEST PREPARATIONS: Motherwort is an exceptionally bitter herb. It should be tinctured fresh. Alternatively, it can be dried for encapsulation or tea, blended with aromatic and pleasing herbs to promote palatability.

HERBAL SUBSTITUTES: Hawthorn (*Crataegus* sp.): cardiovascular | passionflower (*Passiflora incarnata*): anxiety

SAFETY AND PRECAUTIONS

Motherwort is contraindicated for first, second and most of the third trimesters of pregnancy and in instances of postpartum hemorrhage. If you are taking medication for blood pressure, please consult your physician.

LOOK-ALIKES: Mugwort (*Artemisia* sp.)

IDENTIFY & GROW

TYPE OF PLANT: Perennial

HABITAT: Bushy, attractive plant that prefers full sun; often found near waterways and streams

HEIGHT: 3–4' (1–1.3 m)

LEAF: Dark green leaves (sometimes new growth is blushed purple to burgundy) with lighter undersides are deeply divided into three lobes. Each lobe is pointy.

STEM: Square, bristle-y

FLOWER: Pale pink, purple or blue flowers are arranged in whorls up the central stem and typically bloom throughout the summer months.

GROWING INFORMATION: Seeds can be sown directly in the fall, or cold stratified for spring sowing. Seeds and growing plants should be well watered. As a member of the mint family, take steps to control its spread with containers or raised beds.

FORAGE OR GROW? Depending on your area, motherwort may be difficult to find in the wild. Due to ease of cultivation, this is an herb to grow.

BEST HARVEST PRACTICES

FLOWERING TOP HARVEST WINDOW: Early to mid-summer

The flowering tops of motherwort are best harvested when in full bloom. Some people may find the bristle-y stems and leaves irritating to their skin.

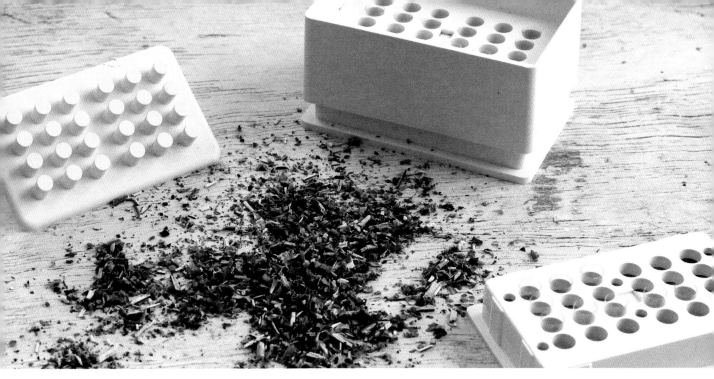

LIONHEARTED MOTHERWORT CAPSULES

Motherwort is a stellar herb for cardiovascular health while also reducing anxiety and nervousness. But it is so very, very bitter that some people cannot tolerate a tea or tincture made from this herb. This is an instance where making capsules is one of the best options for enjoying the benefits of motherwort.

YIELD: 120 capsules

ADULT DOSE: 1–2 capsules, 3 times daily

CHILDREN'S DOSE: While motherwort is safe for children, we generally do not see the need for anxiolytic herbs with young people. If your child is showing signs of anxiety or panic, please consult your physician.

INGREDIENTS

1 oz (28 g) dried motherwort

120 "00" capsules

INSTRUCTIONS

Using a dedicated coffee/spice grinder or a mortar and pestle, grind the motherwort to a fine powder. Using a capsule making tool or filling by hand, pack the motherwort powder into the long end of the capsule and cap tightly. Store in an airtight container in a cool, dark place. Use within 1 year.

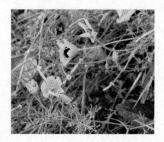

CALIFORNIA POPPY

OTHER COMMON NAMES: poppy, golden poppy, golden cup

LATIN NAME: *Eschscholzia californica*

HERBAL ENERGETICS: cool/dry

THERAPEUTIC ACTIONS: analgesic, anti-inflammatory, antispasmodic, anxiolytic, diaphoretic, diuretic, nervine, sedative

PARTS USED: ariel parts (flower, stem and leaf)

HERBAL MONOGRAPH

I was very excited to learn of the medicinal qualities of California poppy early in my herbal education. To further learn that it is a safe and effective pain reliever and relaxant was even more exciting. While effective for all sorts of pain, California poppy is uniquely well suited to address nerve pain and irritation.

To understand the benefits of California poppy, one must understand the importance of quality sleep and rest. California poppy is a veritable cocktail of pain-relieving and mildly sedating constituents which ameliorate discomfort and restlessness. Essentially, poppy helps to wash away the troubles that hinder restorative sleep so that one can wake up rejuvenated the next morning.

I have found California poppy to be a reliable herb for those with fibromyalgia, migraines, neuralgia and restless legs syndrome. Additionally, those with busy, anxious minds that find themselves pouring over the next day's to-do list can find great relief in small doses of this herb. Some herbalists consider this herb to alleviate some of the agitation and pain associated with acute drug and alcohol withdrawal. It should be noted that while this herb is in the same plant family as the opium poppy, it does not contain any trace of opium and is not a narcotic. It is thought that California poppy acts on the same brain receptors as the more powerful members of the family, fooling the brain into satiety and increasing one's sense of well-being.

California poppy is an excellent remedy for insomnia, promoting a restful night's sleep without being habit forming or leaving one feeling "hazy" upon interrupted sleep. It is also ideal for those that find other sleep-inducing herbs such as valerian or hops objectionable due to odor.

BEST PREPARATIONS: California poppy can be tinctured or dried and added to tea blends. The flower is edible and can be tossed into salads for a colorful addition.

HERBAL SUBSTITUTES: Kava kava (*Piper methysticum*) | valerian (*Valeriana offinalis*)

SAFETY AND PRECAUTIONS

Do not take with other sleep aids or respiratory suppressants, and avoid large doses. If you are pregnant, nursing or taking prescription medication, please consult your physician before taking this or any other herb.

LOOK-ALIKES: Yellow horn poppy (*Glaucium flavum*) TOXIC ROOT, buttercup and other anemones (part of the Ranunculaceae family) VARYING TOXICITY

IDENTIFY & GROW

TYPE OF PLANT: Perennial. This very prolific plant may set seed and produce another flowering plant in the same season, acting as an annual in certain conditions.

HABITAT: California poppies like full sun and well-drained soils. They are often found on roadsides and the edges of cultivated fields and gardens.

HEIGHT: 4–12" (10–30 cm)

LEAF: Alternate, compound, feathery, blue-green leaves

STEM: Erect, branching

FLOWER: Four large petals in shades of yellow and orange with many stamens

GROWING INFORMATION: Sow poppy seeds directly in early spring, covering with a thin layer of light soil. Seeds generally germinate in 10 to 15 days. Do not transplant seedlings, as they prefer not to be disturbed.

FORAGE OR GROW? California residents be warned: It is illegal to gather wild California poppy, so in order to use this botanical you must grow it. It is an attractive and carefree plant once established. For residents of unrestricted states, foraging and growing are both great options.

BEST HARVEST PRACTICES

FLOWER HARVEST WINDOW: Summer

Harvest aerial parts after the morning dew has dried; tincture fresh or dry quickly for teas and infusions.

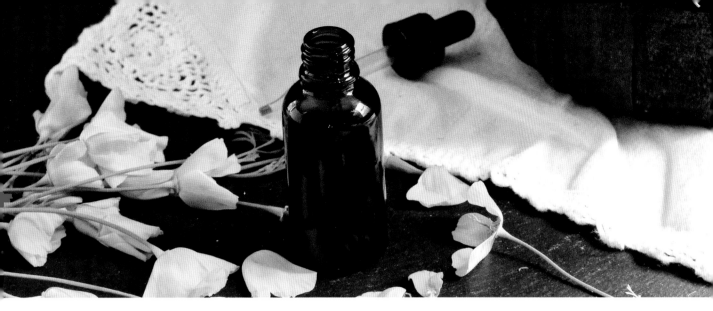

CALIFORNIA POPPY TINCTURE FOR RESTLESSNESS

Insomnia is the pits. And there is more than one kind of insomnia. There is the "I'm just not sleepy" insomnia, and then there is the "I'm exhausted but my mind and body refuse to let me sleep" insomnia. While the former is obnoxious when it rears its pesky head, it is the latter that tends to gnaw away at our well-being at an alarmingly fast rate. This tincture is formulated for those whose bodies and minds are refusing to relax. From herky-jerky legs to anxious and monkey-brained minds, this tincture deploys the gentle-but-effective forces of California poppy, alongside Saint John's wort and lemon balm to lull one into a deep and restful slumber.

The three herbs included in this recipe generally are in peak season at approximately the same time. Please note that the use of Saint John's wort may not be advisable if you are taking certain medications (see page 117) or for administration to children. If you need to avoid Saint John's wort, increase the California poppy accordingly.

YIELD: 1 pint (480 ml)

ADULT DOSE: 1–2 droppers full (1.5–3 ml) in a small glass of water before bedtime

CHILD'S DOSE, AGES 6–12: ½–1 dropper full (0.75–1.5 ml) in a small glass of water before bedtime

NOT RECOMMENDED FOR CHILDREN UNDER THE AGE OF 6.

INGREDIENTS

2 cups (480 ml) 100 proof spirits (vodka recommended)

1 cup (50 g) fresh California poppy flower and leaf, chopped

¼ cup (13 g) fresh Saint John's wort flower tops

¼ cup (13 g) fresh lemon balm leaves, chopped

INSTRUCTIONS

Combine the spirits, poppy, Saint John's wort and lemon balm in a jar with a tight-fitting lid. Infuse for at least 6 weeks. After the infusion is complete, strain the tincture through two layers of cheese cloth or muslin, squeezing to remove as much liquid as possible. Discard the spent plant material in the compost and bottle the tincture in an amber glass master bottle or individual 1- or 2-ounce (30- or 60-ml) bottles. Use within 1 year.

MUGWORT

OTHER COMMON NAMES: artemis herb, felon herb, Saint John's girdle (not to be confused with *Hypericum perforatum*), witches herb, sailor's tobacco

LATIN NAME: *Artemisia vulgaris, A. douglasiana, A. ludoviciana*

HERBAL ENERGETICS: warm/cool/dry

THERAPEUTIC ACTIONS: anthelmintic, antispasmodic, astringent, diaphoretic, digestive, diuretic, emmenagogue, expectorant, nervine, oneirogen (dream enhancer), sedative, tonic, uterine stimulant

PARTS USED: leaves, flowering tops

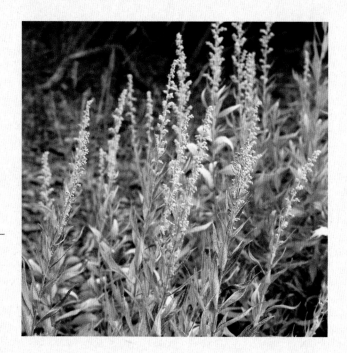

HERBAL MONOGRAPH

At risk of sounding like I am banging the hippie-woo-woo drum, mugwort called to me a few years back. My husband, kids and I were hiking through the dense woods to our favorite swimming and fishing area along the river. Still in the dappled shade of the cottonwoods, along the edge of the wood, my eye spied the characteristic tridented leaf of *Artemisia vulgaris* with the silvery underside in a thicket of blackberries, nettle and other much more abundant plant matter. This habitat is marginal for mugwort at best, and the fact that there were only a few puny, spindly stocks was proof of that fact. I resolved to leave the stand alone, as I could not ethically harvest from such a tiny patch. A little disheartened, I carried on toward the river. And to a rolling sea of coastal mugwort, *A. douglasiana*, along the riverbanks. If you show your restraint and appreciation to the plant world, she often will reward you handsomely.

Among its many virtues, mugwort is perhaps known for one curious feature—its ability to promote vivid, if not lucid, dreams. Perhaps owing to the constituent thujone—which is present in much larger amounts in the notorious, possibly psychedelic, absinthe—mugwort has long been fingered as an herbal tool to encourage visions. Mugwort is sometimes referred to as the "traveler's herb," which may be referencing the more metaphorical meaning of the word "traveler" as much as it refers to alleviating traveling complaints such as fatigue and upset stomach. While there are some reports of mugwort inducing nightmares, that is merely anecdotal, and ethnobotanically speaking, many Native American cultures used mugwort as protection against spirits. While there is no scientific evidence to support the association between mugwort and lucid/vivid dreams, moderate use of the herb tends to increase dream recall in its users.

As a uterine stimulant, mugwort has a long tradition as a women's herb. Mugwort facilitates blood flow to the pelvic region, eliminating the feeling of fullness and bringing on a delayed menses. It is thought to relieve monthly menstrual cramps and soothe labor pains. Although there are some older sources suggesting mugwort in the case of threatened miscarriage, I think that this is a case in which modern wisdom should prevail and mugwort should be avoided during pregnancy. Do not use during labor unless under the guidance and care of an experienced midwife trained in herbs.

Mugwort is also considered an excellent digestive aid. It can stimulate the flow of digestive juices and reduce bloating and after-meal nausea. With a flavor like sage, it can be used culinarily as well as medicinally. In fact, mugwort has been used as a bittering agent for beer making for many centuries. Additionally, this botanical has anthelmintic action, helping to rid the digestive tract of internal parasites.

BEST PREPARATIONS: Mugwort can be tinctured from fresh or dried plant material. Teas and infusions can be prepared from the dry herb; it is suggested to keep your infusing vessel covered to preserve mugwort's volatile oils. Mugwort can also be used as a tobacco substitute in smoking blends or crafted into incense or smudge sticks.

Mugwort is an intense culinary herb with a flavor similar to sage. It is particularly excellent when used to flavor fattier birds such as goose and duck, and it pairs with sweeter vegetables such as winter squash, sweet potatoes and parsnips.

HERBAL SUBSTITUTES: Sage (*Salvia officinalis*): digestive, diaphoretic | kava kava (*Piper methysticum*): dreamwork

SAFETY AND PRECAUTIONS

If you are pregnant, nursing or taking prescription medication, please consult your physician before taking this or any other herb.

LOOK-ALIKES: Wormwood (*Artemisia absinthium*)

IDENTIFY & GROW

TYPE OF PLANT: Perennial

HABITAT: Mugwort prefers full sun to light shade in deep, evenly moist soils. This botanical is often found by streams, rivers and gravel bars.

HEIGHT: 3–6' (1–2 m) depending on species

LEAF: Varies somewhat between species. Leaves are arranged alternately and get smaller and narrower as they rise up the stem. Leaves resemble a trident (some species being more finely cut, and each lobe is irregularly toothed). The upper side of the leaves is green and hairless, while the underside is downy and quite silver-gray by comparison. Very strong sage-like aroma.

STEM: Strong stems that are hairless until the flowering tops

FLOWER: Nondescript panicles of yellowish-green to rust colored flowers at the top of stems; characteristic sage fragrance

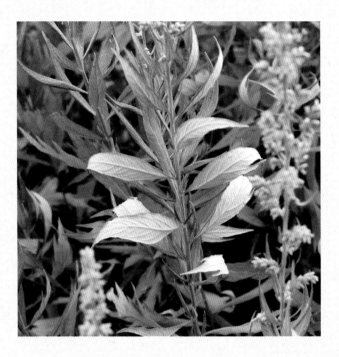

GROWING INFORMATION: Sow seeds directly into damp peat moss in fall or cold stratify for 2 to 4 weeks for early spring germination. Plant in full sun in well-drained soils with ample water supply. Mugwort will tolerate some drought, but it thrives with decent moisture

FORAGE OR GROW? The various species of mugwort are fairly easy to locate in the wild landscape and tend to flourish given the right conditions, making it an easy botanical to forage. It is also a very attractive plant (particularly *A. ludoviciana*), with its green and silver foliage making a beautiful foil for more colorful plants.

BEST HARVEST PRACTICES
LEAF AND FLOWERING TOP HARVEST WINDOW: Mid-summer

Mugwort is ideally harvested at or near the time of flowering to maximize its volatile oil content.

MUGWORT & LAVENDER SMUDGE STICKS FOR PLEASANT DREAMS

Smudging, the burning of tightly bound bundles of dried herbs, is observed in a number of different cultures and traditions throughout the world. Mugwort and lavender are both highly aromatic and produce a smoke with a relaxing aroma. Burned before bedtime, this smudge will promote a restful, dream-filled sleep.

These instructions make for a small- to medium-sized stick. You can add more herbal sprigs for a fuller stick, if you prefer.

NOTE: Burn the smudge stick on a heatproof surface, such as a ceramic plate or bowl. For safety reasons, do not leave the smudge to burn unattended or fall asleep when burning a smudge.

YIELD: 1 stick

INGREDIENTS

5 sprigs of fresh mugwort

1 sprig of fresh lavender

Cotton thread

INSTRUCTIONS

Gather the fresh herbs into tight bundles about 6-inches (15-cm) long and no bigger than 1 inch (2.5 cm) in diameter. Using a crisscross pattern, secure the bundle with thread down the length of the herbs. Tie off tightly. To dry, either place the bundles in a dehydrator or hang to dry thoroughly. Store in a sealed container in a cool, dark place. Use within 1 year.

To use, using a lighter or a wooden match, light one end of the smudge and allow a strong flame to develop. This may take a few seconds or upwards of a minute depending on the compactness and residual moisture content of your smudge stick. Once the flame is hot and well established, gently blow out the flame and place the smudge in or on a heatproof vessel to smolder and release its aromatic smoke.

Not recommended for use with children.

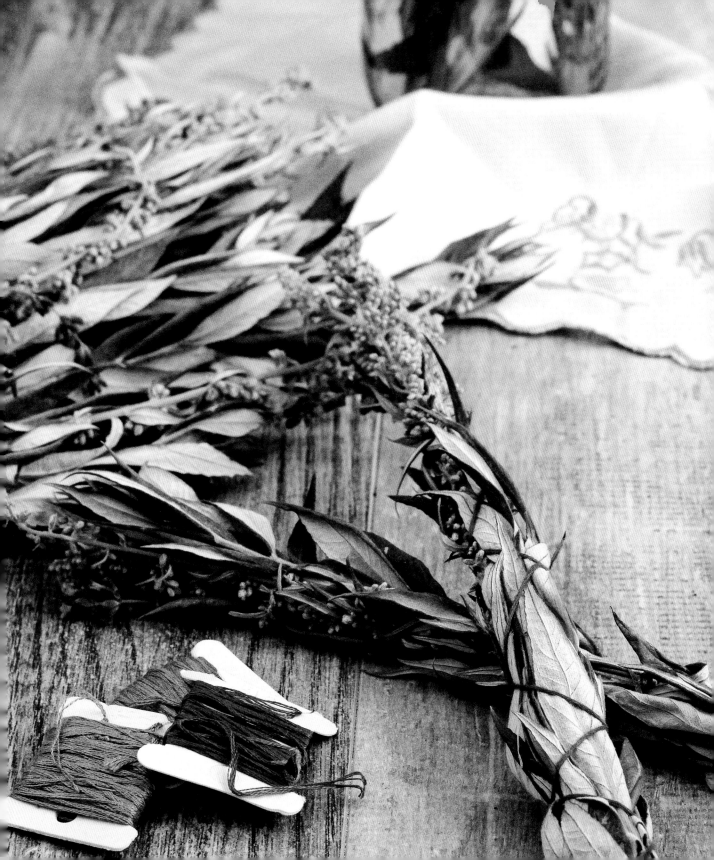

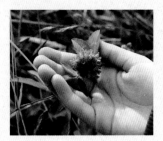

RED CLOVER

OTHER COMMON NAMES: cow clover, tripata

LATIN NAME: *Trifolium pratense*

HERBAL ENERGETICS: cool/neutral

THERAPEUTIC ACTIONS: alterative, antiallergenic, anti-inflammatory, antineoplastic, antioxidant, antispasmodic, cardiovascular, emmenagogue, hepatic, lymphatic, nutritive,

PARTS USED: leaf, flowering tops

HERBAL MONOGRAPH

As a farmer, you rarely hit the trifecta of pasture weeds: something that grows prolifically, something that does positive things for the soil and something that is safe and nutritious for your grazing animals. As an herbalist, you are rarely championing a botanical that farmers love. But with red clover, your bases are covered.

All things considered, red clover is just a powerhouse herb. It is abundantly nutritious and offers a whole host of medicinal benefits. It is most often thought of as an herb for women's health due to its high quantity of isoflavones, as well as calcium and magnesium. As a nutritive tonic for the reproductive organs, it is often suggested for peri-menopause and menopausal symptoms such as hot flashes, night sweats, mild depression, mood changes and vaginal dryness. It has been suggested for menstrual cramps. Red clover is also called for when there are complaints of ovarian cysts, uterine fibroids and hard fibrous breast tissue. There is also mounting clinical evidence to support the herb's use in the prevention of bone loss contributing to osteoporosis. While there has been some controversy about whether red clover is appropriate for those with a family history of estrogen-dependent cancers, a 2008 study of over 400 women, ages 35 to 70, showed no increase in adverse effects when compared to placebo. Not limited to concerns of women's health, it is also suggested for prostate concerns and swollen, enflamed testicles.

Red clover is also an outstanding herb for the cardiovascular system. Considered a blood "purifier" in the herbal community, this herb has been shown to inhibit the formation of plaque on arterial walls and reduce inflammation, according to a 2010 study. Additionally, these alterative "purification properties" often benefit those suffering with acne, eczema, psoriasis and other skin irritations. As a noteworthy lymphatic, red clover is considered in cases of edema and hardened, sore lymph nodes.

BEST PREPARATIONS: Red clover is best extracted in water. Extended infusion time of 4 to 12 hours is suggested to extract the nutritive value of this plant.

HERBAL SUBSTITUTES: Alfalfa (*Medicago sativa*): nutritive | cleaver (*Galium aparine*): lymphatic

SAFETY AND PRECAUTIONS

Do not use red clover when pregnant or nursing due to its phyto-estrogen content. Please consult your physician before using this herb if you or your family have a history of estrogen dependent cancers.

LOOK-ALIKES: White clover (*Trifolium repens*), crimson clover (*Trifolium incarnatum*)

IDENTIFY & GROW

TYPE OF PLANT: Annual (sometimes perennial in northern climates)

HABITAT: Red clover likes part to full sun with moist but well-drained soil. Grows particularly well in rich soil.

HEIGHT: 12–36" (30–90 cm)

LEAF: Stem arises from a compound leaf with groupings (1 to 3) of 3 oval leaflets with a white or pale green V.

STEM: Hollow, hairy stems

FLOWER: Approximately 1" (2.5-cm) pink flower head with many small tubular flowers. May be white at base.

GROWING INFORMATION: Seed can be broadcast before the last frost or in early spring in moist but not damp soils to reap multiple summer harvests.

FORAGE OR GROW? Red clover is easy to forage, but it does tend to grow in areas of potential waste runoff and near farms that may use chemical fertilizers, pesticides and herbicides. I would encourage readers to grow red clover.

BEST HARVEST PRACTICES

FLOWER HARVEST WINDOW: Early to mid-summer

Harvest the upper leaves and flowering tops of red clover throughout the season, after any morning dew has dried. Red clover can be dried whole, but special care should be taken to see that they are fully dried before storage as they are very dense. I personally prefer to pull the small individual flowers off prior to drying to ensure a good result.

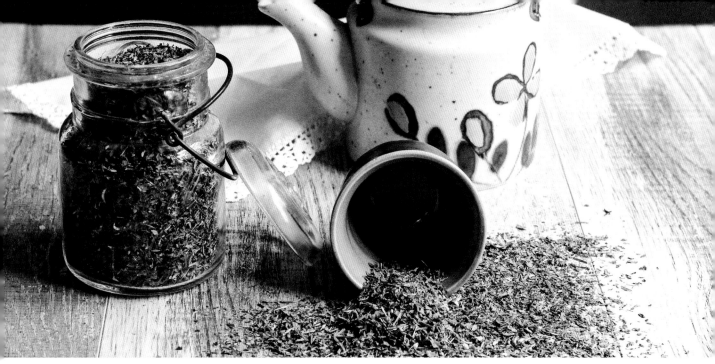

NOURISHING RED CLOVER HERBAL INFUSION FOR MENOPAUSAL SUPPORT

Red clover, red clover—send relief from hot flashes and mood swings on over! Also send all the vital nutrients to support bone health during and after menopause. Red clover and catmint combine in this delicious herbal tea to promote an even keel and all over coolness, especially when night sweats and hot flashes are a major complaint. This tea is especially lovely iced, sipped as a nourishing herbal infusion throughout the day.

YIELD: 4 cups (100 g) of dry blend

ADULT DOSE: 16–32 oz (475–950 ml) sipped throughout the day

INGREDIENTS

3 cups (75 g) dried red clover blossom and leaf

1 cup (25 g) dried catmint

INSTRUCTIONS

Combine the herbs, and store in a jar with a tight-fitting lid in a cool, dark place.

To prepare the infusion: Add 2 to 3 tablespoons (3 to 5 g) of the herbal blend to a quart-sized (1-L) jar. Fill the jar with water just off the boil. Allow the jar to cool for at least 30 minutes, then move the jar to the refrigerator to cool and infuse for 6 to 12 hours. After infusing, strain the infusion and pour over ice. Store unused infusion in the refrigerator and use within 48 hours. Use the dried herbal blend within 1 year.

BLACK WALNUT

OTHER COMMON NAMES: American walnut, eastern walnut

LATIN NAME: *Juglans nigra*

HERBAL ENERGETICS: cool/dry

THERAPEUTIC ACTIONS: anti-inflammatory, antimicrobial, antioxidant, antiparasitic, astringent, cholagogue, digestive, hypotensive, nutritive (nut), vulnerary

PARTS USED: green hull, nut (edible)

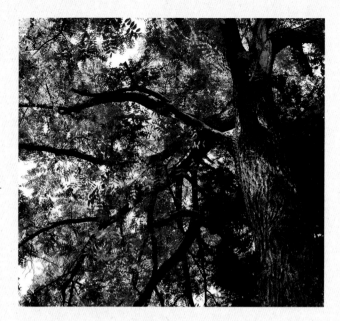

HERBAL MONOGRAPH

I find that client compliance when using herbal medicine is best when the herb being used is something that they know and recognize. It takes the fear-of-the-unknown quotient down a few notches, priming the body for healing, reinforced by positive thinking. Black walnuts are the wilder and wilier cousin to the large and stately English walnut. A tasty and nutritious nut in a well-fortified shell, black walnuts are often cast aside for culinary purposes in favor of the meatier English varieties. But wild foodies and herbalists know that black walnuts are an abundant gift from nature—offering food and medicine to those unafraid of contributing a little effort. Furthermore, black walnut hulls are an excellent remedy for the things that make us most squeamish—fungal and parasitic infections.

The very thought of internal parasites usually gives people the creeps. Truth be told, even after farming and taking extensive pathology courses with GRAPHIC texts, the thought of "worms" makes me shudder. But the simple fact of the matter is if you have ever handled pets or livestock, swam in or accidentally drank suspect water, ate mishandled food or even walked barefoot through the lawn, chances are you have either experienced or had a near miss with a parasitic infection. Signs of internal parasites include bloating, nausea, diarrhea, abdominal pain, fatigue, weight loss, anemia and, everybody's favorite, anal itching. Black walnut hulls are highly antiparasitic against round, pin and tape worms, aiding in their expulsion.

With one icky subject out of the way, let's address another unlikely candidate for Miss Congeniality in the health concern pageant: fungal infections. Common fungal infections include athlete's foot, ringworm (not caused by parasites as the name suggests), candida (responsible for vaginal yeast infections, oral thrush and diaper rashes), as well as lesser-known complaints like onychomycosis (yellowing of the nailbed) and tinea versicolor (scaly and discolored skin). Again, here we find black walnut to be a powerful aid in the more embarrassing of health concerns.

In an altogether less disturbing subject, black walnut shares many of the same health benefits linked to English walnut and is linked to decreased inflammation and increased cardiovascular health.

BEST PREPARATIONS: Black walnut hulls are very tannic. They can be prepared as teas or infusions, but may be more effective and palatable as a tincture. Salves prepared from black walnut hull–infused oil make exceptional ointments for external complaints.

HERBAL SUBSTITUTES: Wormwood (*Artemisia absinthium*): parasites | chaparral (*Larrea tridentata*): fungus

SAFETY AND PRECAUTIONS

Avoid black walnut use if allergic to walnuts or any other nut. If you are pregnant, nursing or taking prescription medications, please consult your physician before taking this or any other herb.

LOOK-ALIKES: American or white ash (*Fraxinus* sp.), pecan (*Carya illinoinensis*)

IDENTIFY & GROW

❀ **TYPE OF PLANT**: Deciduous tree

❀ **HABITAT**: Black walnut trees prefer full sun and deep, somewhat moist soil.

❀ **HEIGHT**: Aged trees have been recorded at over 100' (30 m)

❀ **LEAF**: 12–24" (30–60-cm) leaves. Leaves are alternate and compound with 11 or more leaflets.

❀ **TRUNK**: Dark brown, deeply furrowed bark

❀ **NUT**: Slightly smaller than a golf ball, green fruits appear in early summer. As the nuts mature, the outer hulls wither and darken; the internal shell hardens to protect the walnut "meat."

❀ **GROWING INFORMATION**: Black walnuts can be grown from the nut, but this will take a number of years to mature. Buy young organic trees from a reputable nursery and plant in a sunny location with deep soils, in a spot not prone to excessive frost.

❀ **FORAGE OR GROW?** Depending on your location, black walnuts may be quite prolific and excellent foraging fare even in an urban setting. A well-established tree provides ample shade and makes an attractive landscape plant.

BEST HARVEST PRACTICES
HULL HARVEST WINDOW: Early fall

Gather walnuts as they fall to the ground in late summer and early fall. Wearing gloves, slough off the outer hull. You may need to use a paring knife to remove more stubborn hulls. Immediately dry or tincture the hull or dry for future use. Wear gloves and protect sustainable surfaces when working with walnuts.

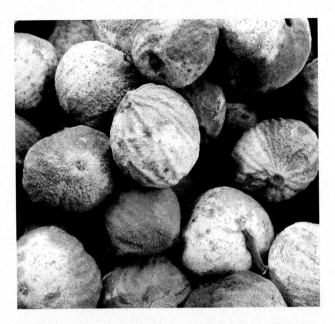

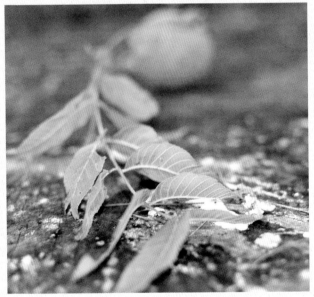

FUNGAL FIGHTING BLACK WALNUT SALVE

As a farmer, I have had the great misfortune to experience a horrifically awful case of ringworm, courtesy of an afflicted calf that was dropped into my care. I literally tried everything—including straight essential oils and over-the-counter and prescription antifungals. Some things would decrease my discomfort, but nothing was getting rid of my embarrassing and unsightly spots. I finally put my (then) newfound herbal knowledge to work and made this salve. It worked like a charm. I was spot-free in a little over a week!

Black walnut, neem oil and a couple powerful antifungal essential oils team up in this salve to deliver some strong antifungal action. While the rest of my recipes will often suggest essential oils as an optional ingredient, here I strongly encourage you to use them. Firstly, because a good neem oil smells a bit of burning tires and garlic, and secondly, because they add further antifungal action to the blend. Black walnut is the star of this blend, but fungal infections such as ringworm, athlete's foot and jock itch deserve to have a holistic fungal fighting league of warriors unleashed on them. This blend delivers just that!

YIELD: approximately 8 ounces (240 ml)

INGREDIENTS

½ cup (55 g) dried black walnut hulls

¾ cup plus 2 tbsp (195 g) coconut oil

2 tbsp (30 ml) neem oil

2–4 tbsp (20–40 g) beeswax pastilles

48 drops geranium essential oil

48 drops oregano essential oil

INSTRUCTIONS

Using the heated oil infusion method (page 12), infuse the black walnut hulls into the coconut and neem oil for 72 hours. After the oil is adequately infused, strain through muslin or cheese cloth. Return the oil to a double boiler, add the beeswax and warm until completely melted. Remove the oil-beeswax mixture from the heat and stir in the essential oils. Pour into individual 2-ounce (60-ml) containers, approximately 4, or other similarly sized jars. Allow to cool completely before putting a lid on the jar. Use within 1 year.

Apply to affected areas as needed until all traces of the complaint have disappeared. Do not use if allergic to walnuts. If you experience hives or respiratory distress, seek immediate medical attention.

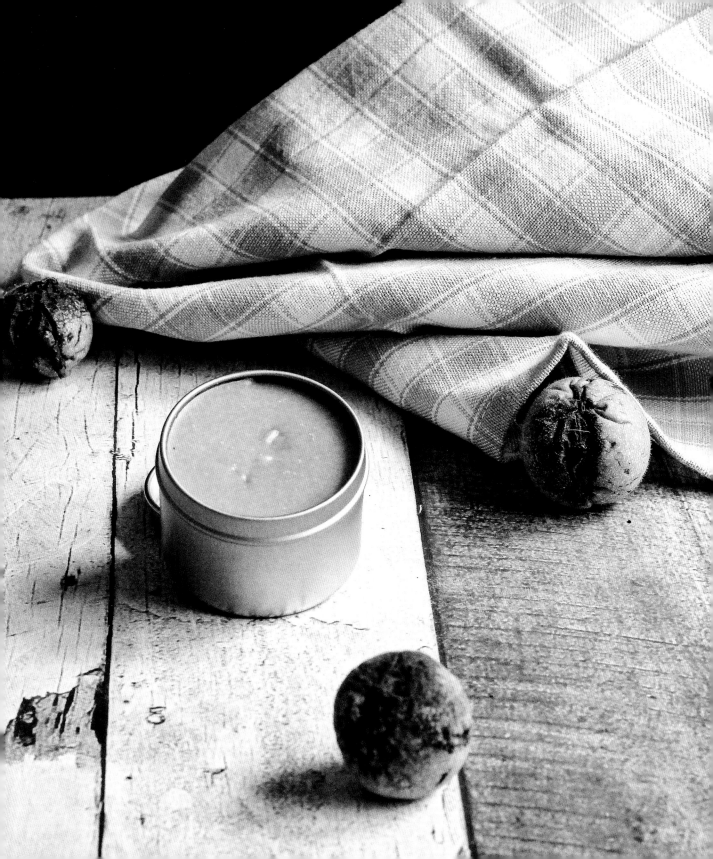

COMMON YARD DAISY

OTHER COMMON NAMES: English daisy, dog daisy, bruisewort, woundwort

LATIN NAME: *Bellis perennis*

HERBAL ENERGETICS: cool /dry (flowers), moist (leaves)

THERAPEUTIC ACTIONS: anti-rheumatic, antispasmodic, antitussive, astringent, demulcent (leaves), digestive, expectorant, febrifuge, laxative (leaves, mild), styptic

PARTS USED: flower, leaves

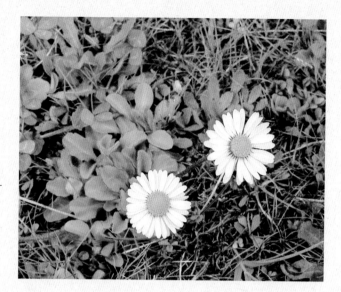

HERBAL MONOGRAPH

These are the blossoms of daisy chains. The flower crowns of school-age children and festival-loving hipsters alike. They are the harbinger of spring—dotting lawns with their cheerful faces, often well before the sunnier dandelions stretch their golden petals upward. Flower folklore weaves stories of the ever-popular rose—who had a splendid party including all the flower world as guests. Except the tiny little daisy—overlooked and unnoticed. Upon learning of the oversight, rose made a grand invitation to the lovely little daisy, causing the wee, shy flower to blush. The common yard daisy is small, delicate, perhaps unassuming—and it is often mowed over without as much as a second thought given to its medicinal virtue. Let's be roses and invite the little daisy to the party.

And for all its diminutive presence, the common lawn daisy is a force to be reckoned with.

I like to say this baby daisy is the poor man's arnica. Or more aptly put, the "don't-live-or-forage-in-sub-Alpine-regions" arnica. But that is a bit long-winded. Its older, colloquial common names shed light on its uses: bruisewort and woundwort (wort means flower or bloom). Ancient documents make mention of this herb being used by the Roman legions to pack wounds and poultice bruises. While the modern-day herbalist might be reluctant to pack a fresh wound with the botanical matter, the common yard daisy can certainly be applied as a poultice over deep tissue bruises as a poultice or infused salve. Supporting its use as a vulnerary herb, a small 2012 study using lab rats demonstrated that use of an ointment containing a fractionated *Bellis perennis* ointment on excision wounds resulted in better wound closure and decrease in scar tissue formation. This gentle daisy is indicated for heavy menstrual flow and obstetric injuries, such as postpartum bleeding, when consumed as an infusion.

The common yard daisy is a notable expectorant, particularly well suited to the evacuation of catarrh—excessive mucus in the throat and nose. It is may also relieve pain and sensation of heat in the throat, making it particularly comforting for a flu accompanied by fever. Daisy can also be useful for normalizing digestive issues, increasing tone of the intestinal wall, decreasing abdominal cramping and promoting regular bowel movements.

BEST PREPARATIONS: The common yard daisy lends itself to a variety of preparations, both topical and internal. A poultice of fresh ground flowers, leaves and a little liquid such as water or witch hazel can be applied to areas of blunt trauma or bruising. The flowers and leaves can also be gathered and dried for infusing in oils for salve making, and for internal applications such as teas, infusions and tinctures.

HERBAL SUBSTITUTES: Arnica (*Arnica montana*): bruising | yarrow (*Achillea millefolium*): bleeding

SAFETY AND PRECAUTIONS

Although a gentle herb, it should be avoided by those with bleeding disorders or on anticoagulant therapies. It should also be avoided by those taking medicinal doses of blood-thinning herbs, such as garlic. Although daisy is indicated for obstetric injury, this should be for acute uses only, such as non-emergent yet heavy postpartum bleeding; otherwise, avoid during pregnancy or while nursing. There are unsubstantiated claims that its use may stunt the growth of a fetus or infant.

LOOK-ALIKES: Other *Bellis* species

IDENTIFY & GROW

🌸 **TYPE OF PLANT**: Perennial

🌸 **HABITAT**: This diminutive daisy is a common lawn "weed" or "pest" growing in areas of sun to part or dappled shade and ample soil moisture. It forms low-growing, dense mats of foliage and blooms in early spring. It is hardy to zone 4, although it may suffer in extended periods of heat and dryness.

🌸 **HEIGHT**: 2–8" (5–20 cm)

🌸 **LEAF**: Forms a basal rosette of oval leaves with irregular serrated margins

🌸 **STEM**: Leafless, hairy stem

🌸 **FLOWER**: White or white-blushed with slender pink bracts radiating from a central yellow capitula. Cultivated varieties of *Bellis perennis* may also be observed in various hues of pink and violet. Note: When identifying members of the Asteraceae (daisy) family, the technical botanical vocabulary is more detailed and specific as the center is the actual "flower," and what we commonly refer to as petals are actually bracts.

🌸 **SEED**: Small oval, without seams or hairs; appearing late summer to fall

🌸 **FORAGE OR GROW?** This is an easy herb to identify and forage. Domesticated cultivars exist, but they are of lesser medicinal value. This is an herb to forage.

BEST HARVEST PRACTICES
FLOWER HARVEST WINDOW: Spring

While this herb is very common in lawns and grassy meadows, always harvest from areas that are free of herbicides, ground pollutants/contaminated runoff and pet urine or feces.

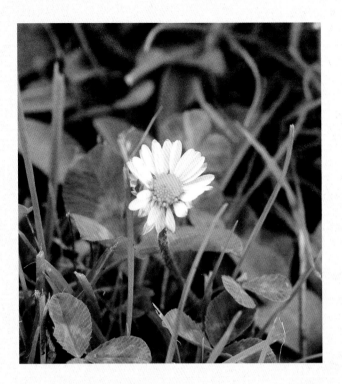

TIP: The common yard daisy is the poor man's arnica. It's a wonderful herb for bruising, sprains, strains, and minor wounds.

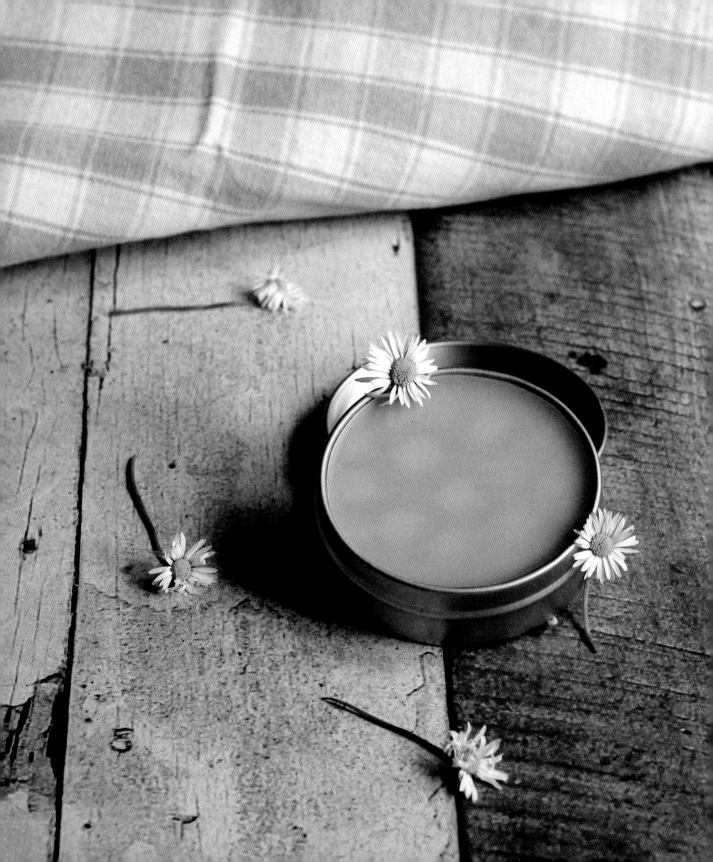

POORMAN'S BRUISE BALM WITH COMMON YARD DAISY

While even armchair herbalists have heard of the anti-bruising action of arnica (which also makes a great substitution if you miss the best harvest window for daisy), not many know of the similar actions of the much more common yard daisy. This little balm is perfect for those minor bruises, bumps, strains and mild sprains of everyday life.

YIELD: approximately 8 ounces (240 ml)

INGREDIENTS

1 cup (240 ml) base oil blend of your choice (I like coconut oil and olive oil)

½ cup (13 g) dried common yard daisy

2–4 tbsp (20–40 g) beeswax pastilles

50 drops helichrysum essential oil (optional)

INSTRUCTIONS

Using the regular or heated oil infusion method (page 12), infuse the daisies into the base oils. After the oil is adequately infused, strain through muslin or cheese cloth.

Return the oil to a double boiler, add the beeswax and warm until completely melted. Remove the oil-beeswax mixture from the heat, and stir in the essential oil if desired. Pour into individual 2-ounce (60-ml) containers, approximately 4, or other similarly sized jars. Allow to cool completely before putting a lid on the container.

Apply to affected areas as needed until bruising and inflammation decrease. Use within 1 year.

PLANTAIN

OTHER COMMON NAMES: ripple grass, snakeweed, English man's foot, psyllium, ribwort

LATIN NAME: *Plantago major, P. lancelota*

HERBAL ENERGETICS: cool/neutral (leaf), moist (seed)

THERAPEUTIC ACTIONS: anti-inflammatory, antimicrobial, anti-obtrusive, astringent, demulcent, diuretic, expectorant, hepatic, nutritive, vulnerary

PARTS USED: leaf, seed

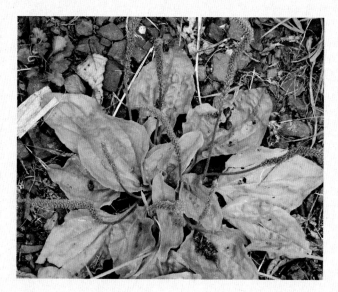

HERBAL MONOGRAPH

Plantain is inevitably an herb that most people have seen, but not given any thought to. Its deeply veined leaves often blend in with blades of grass (especially the narrow leaved variety), and the only real sign that there is something different afoot is when the slender flower stalk with its cone-shaped plume rises above the denser vegetation below. It is the proverbial wallflower of the herbal medicine world. It is simply not going to jump right out and snag your attention with flowers, thorns or flashy foliage. Plantain has a quiet, dutiful demeanor, and it is an indispensable plant ally for oh-so-many reasons.

What plantain lacks in botanical pizzazz, it makes up for in its abundant medicinal virtues. Plantain is a soft-spoken heroine that doesn't ask for thanks but deserves the recognition.

If you had to boil down the medicinal attributes of plantain, the reductionist outcome would be that it is a drawing herb. We use the leaf to draw out heat, infection, venom, phlegm, excess fluid and more. Plantain is the friend that comes over to your house when you are overwhelmed by a mess and knows exactly what needs to be discarded. It removes what is out of place and repairs all the physical damage it's exposed to. It is my favorite herb for drawing forth splinters, stickers and stingers that are deep in the skin, making it perfect for little ones who tremble with fear at the sight of tweezers or needles used for extraction. It is also extremely soothing and provides itch relief for bug bites and rashes. Older texts refer to its use with snake and rabid dog bites—though please consider this but an herbal first aid on

your way to getting immediate medical attention, rather than an alternative to conventional care.

Its gentle, yet effective, astringent properties make plantain an excellent herb for cough, cold symptoms and seasonal allergies. Weepy, watery eyes and runny noses seem to respond very well to plantain, as do thick, hot, productive coughs and swollen, painful lymph nodes. Other indications point to its use to draw infection from oral abscess of the teeth and gums. This herb can also bring tremendous relief to hemorrhoids, applied as a poultice or as a sitz bath.

Plantain use extends to the fiber-rich seeds, known as psyllium. Psyllium is commonly sold as a fiber supplement and highly effective for complaints of the lower bowel, such as constipation, colitis, Crohn's, enteritis and dysentery. Additionally, numerous studies have found that the seeds help reduce cholesterol levels and hyperlipidemia, as well as hyperglycemia, while having net positive effects on the cardiovascular system.

> **NOTE:** The *Plantago* herb, commonly known as plantain, is not nor has any relation to the plantain of the banana family (*Musa* spp.).

BEST PREPARATIONS: This is an herb that can be used in a variety of ways. Teas, tinctures and oil infusions for salve making are popular methods of preparation. Perhaps one of the simplest methods of use is the "spit poultice"—chewed leaves applied to spots of irritation and heat. If this method feels a bit too unsanitary, a poultice prepared with water or a juicing of the leaves may be more appropriate. Due to its vulnerary nature, it is ideal for use on cuts and scrapes—especially those incurred while wrangling blackberries as my experience would suggest!

Psyllium seeds can be soaked in liquids and/or added to smoothies.

HERBAL SUBSTITUTES: Common yard daisy (*Bellis perenis*)

SAFETY AND PRECAUTIONS
This herb is widely regarded as safe. If pregnant, nursing or taking prescription medication, please consult with your physician before taking this or any other herb. Note: Some people with certain bowel conditions should avoid fibers such as psyllium.

LOOK-ALIKES: Hosta (*Hosta* spp.)

IDENTIFY & GROW

🌸 **TYPE OF PLANT:** Perennial

🌸 **HABITAT:** Plantain is often in lawns and pastures where the water is plentiful, but not soggy.

🌸 **HEIGHT:** 4–6" (10–15 cm)

🌸 **LEAF:** Depending on the particular species, leaves can be long, lance-shaped (*P. lancelota*) or more rounded with a pointed tip resembling a small hosta leaf (*P. major*). Plantago leaves are deeply ribbed and form a basal rosette.

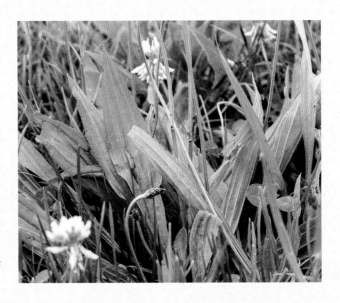

🌸 **FLOWER/SEED:** Forms an upright spike topped with a brown cone with small white, inconspicuous flowers

🌸 **GROWING INFORMATION:** It is altogether likely that you are, in fact, currently growing plantain in your yard. If not, seeds can be sown in the spring in a sunny to part-shade location that will receive frequent watering but has well-drained soil. Cold stratification may contribute to good germination rates.

🌸 **FORAGE OR GROW?** Due to the relative ease in which plantain grows in the yard, this is an herb to forage.

BEST HARVEST PRACTICES
HARVEST WINDOW: Early spring through fall

Ensure that you are harvesting plantain from herbicide-, pesticide-, fertilizer-, pet waste–free areas. The herb can be used fresh or dried quickly for future use and oil infusions.

PLANTAIN POULTICE FOR PULLING SPLINTERS, STINGERS & OTHER OFFENDERS

This spectacularly easy preparation is so effective (and safe) that everybody needs to know about it. Plantain grows virtually anywhere and is so easy to identify—it makes for first aid on the fly when needed. This is another method where there is no exact measurement. Just make a paste of chopped (or even chewed, in a pinch) plantain and a tiny bit of water, and apply to an affected area (splinters, stingers, bug bites, etc.) for quick relief!

It is easy to fall into the trap of "more is better," but sometimes the best remedy is the simplest and, more importantly, the one that is immediately available to you. For example, if you are spending an afternoon at the park and one of you children gets stung, chances are you won't have a drawing salve with you in that moment of need. BUT, the likelihood of there being some plantain growing nearby is great. The best medicine is the one you have access to! It is vital to learn these simple, simple remedies, because there will be a time in your life when you need them! For additional cooling relief of inflamed areas, substitute aloe in place of water to reduce redness and irritation.

This remedy is safe for adults and children.

YIELD: varies

INGREDIENTS

Fresh plantain

Water, aloe or the gel exudate expressed from the bottom of a dock leaf stem

INSTRUCTIONS

Make a thick paste of finely chopped or chewed plantain and a small amount of water. You'll want a texture like pesto. Smear on affected areas. If it dries and irritation persists, reapply as necessary. Use immediately.

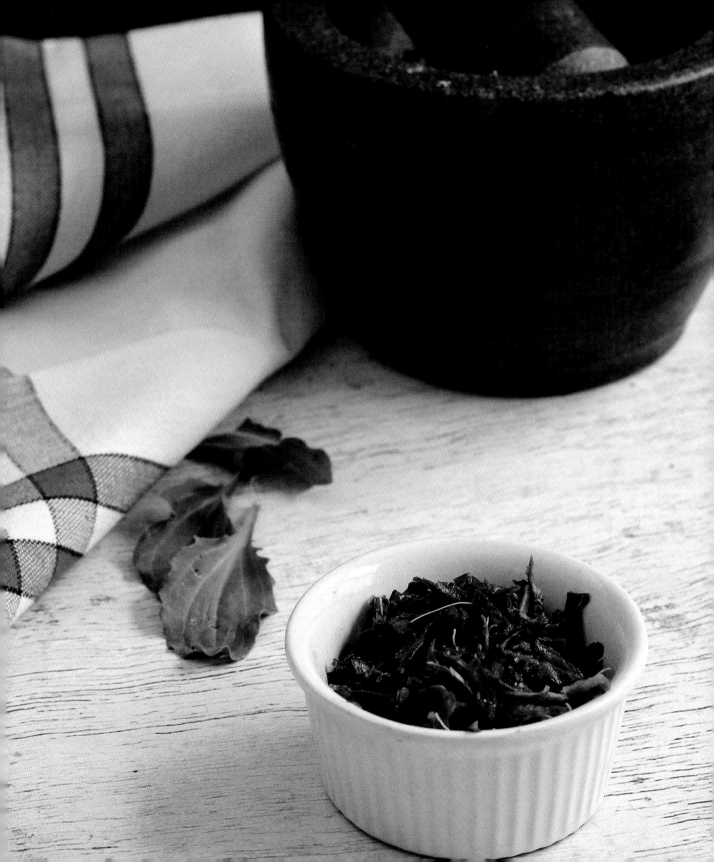

SAINT JOHN'S WORT

OTHER COMMON NAMES: Saint Joan's wort, Touch and Heal, Goatsweed, scare-devil, Klamath Weed, balm of warriors wound, Tipton weed, Amber, rose of Sharon (a shared named with a mallow family botanical)

LATIN NAME: *Hypericum perforatum*

HERBAL ENERGETICS: cool/dry

THERAPEUTIC ACTIONS: alterative, analgesic, antibacterial, antidepressant, anti-inflammatory, antispasmodic, antiviral, astringent, hepatic, nervine, sedative, tropho-restorative, vulnerary

PARTS USED: aerial parts

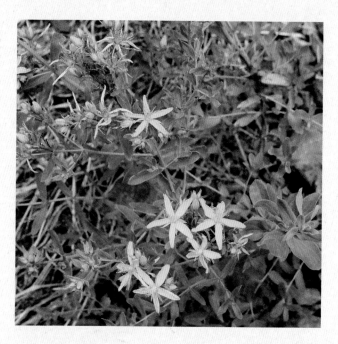

HERBAL MONOGRAPH

Saint John's wort. Undoubtedly you have heard of it. It is the herb for depression, right?

"The herb for depression" is a common statement that makes many herbalists cringe. Firstly, the statement is so singular and myopic in its scope. And secondly, any decent herbalist and anybody that has ever suffered from depression knows that there is no "one size fits all" cure for the darkness that sometimes shadows our souls. Furthermore, pigeonholing this herb to depression-related applications is the type of false heroic behavior that hurts more than it helps the alternative, naturalistic health movement.

Saint John's wort is so much more than an herb for depression. It is an herb for the whole body and soul.

I encourage readers to think of Saint John's wort as an herb for bodily systems, rather than an herb for bodily symptoms. It is a restorative herb. It restores the nervous system. It restores the immune system. It restores the integumentary (skin) system. It is the visionary mechanic of the herbal world—repairing and replenishing the damaged and worn parts of our personal "vehicle" so that we can move through life again.

The exact mechanism by which Saint John's wort alters depressive states is largely unknown, with some scientists pointing to its ability to normalize brain serotonin levels. Herbalists often see Saint John's wort through a different lens, one that operates from a theory of wholism. Translation: Increase the health and function of all organ systems and the whole being benefits, physically as well as emotionally. This is especially well observed with the effects of St. John's wort on the nervous system.

Saint John's wort is thought to be deeply connected to the nerves, organs and muscles of the solar plexus area. It is in this solar plexus area that the fibers of the vagus nerve branch out and start "wandering" the abdominal cavity. Stay with me while I draw a connection between the vagus nerve and the use of Saint John's wort. The vagus nerve is linked to your gut "instinct"—the afferent fibers sending signals to the brain—and your body's digestive response to stress—the efferent fibers sending signals from the brain to the gut. The vagus nerve intrinsically "knows" the difference between innate and conditioned, or learned, fears. A study of rats with artificially severed vagus nerves demonstrated that the rats had a decreased response to innate fears, while having an increased, prolonged response to conditioned fears. This suggests that the suboptimal vagus nerve conditions contribute to unbalanced fear responses. Here is where I propose that Saint John's wort serves its very important role. This botanical is a tropho-restorative with a strong affinity for the nervous system. It is a well-regarded herb in the holistic community for use with complaints of the nervous system. It stands to reason that by nourishing and protecting the vagus nerve, Saint John's wort may have a normalizing effect on fear—or more specifically on anxiety. There is even scientific evidence showing that this herb improves synaptic response. By conjecture, this herb is less suited for gloom-and-doom style depression, but more tailor-made for those with mutinous anxiety that can quite literally be felt in the gut. Saint John's wort is for those that become sick with worry, the "what if-ers," the perpetual "future trippers" and those that receive evacuation orders from their digestive system at the hint of trouble to come.

Similarly, Saint John's wort is a premier herb for nerve pain. Nerve pain has a certain electric, instantaneous quality to it that is hard to describe until you have experienced it yourself. It can be crippling. Types of nerve pain include sciatica, shingles and neuropathy. Internal and external use of St. John's wort is known to diminish nerve pain for many users. Furthermore, Saint John's wort, in combination with lemon balm perhaps, is one of the herbs most ideally suited to the pain associated with shingles, while also serving to provide further benefit with its antiviral properties.

Not only is Saint John's wort a mender of nerve fibers and a supporter of good mental health, but it is also an herb that promotes healthy liver function by enhancing the liver's natural detoxification process. This is of particular relevance where we see suppressed liver functionality, such as with recovery from alcohol addiction, as well as estrogen dominance as observed with marked premenstrual syndrome (PMS) symptoms. Saint John's wort hastens the P450 metabolic pathway, which expedites the liver's normal detoxification process. Do note that this may be desirable in instances of liver congestion, but the speedy metabolic effect can reduce the efficacy of some medications, such as statins and oral contraception.

No discussion of Saint John's wort is complete with speaking to its powerful first aid actions. As some of the common names suggest, this herb offers profound wound-healing benefits. Being a sound antibacterial and a strong vulnerary, Saint John's wort helps to stave off infection and weave the fabric of the skin back together. Some herbalists suggest that internal use of this herb will help promote the repair of nerve to deep tissue cuts and encourage nerve regrowth where an amputated limb has been reattached. Less dramatically, it is an herb that ameliorates bruising and relieves the pain and inflammation resulting from a sunburn.

BEST PREPARATIONS: Saint John's wort is an herb that is considered its most potent when used fresh. The fresh leaves and flowering tops exude a rich red juice that imparts its color into any menstruum to which it is introduced. It can be tinctured fresh in alcohol; I prefer to wilt freshly harvested Saint John's wort before infusing in oil in order to drive out a small amount of moisture, then cover the jar or vessel with thin cloth to promote continued moisture evaporation. Infused oils are good for massage and for salve making. The dried herb is still very suitable for use, although some, but not all, would argue that it is slightly less efficacious. Personally, I prefer to use the herb fresh, but I am by no means deterred from a project or remedy when only dried herb is available. The dried herb can be ground to powder and encapsulated, a remedy especially appropriate for those opposed to an alcohol-based tincture.

HERBAL SUBSTITUTES: Lion's mane (*Hericium erinaceus*): nerve restorative | passionflower (*Passiflora incarnata*): anxiety

SAFETY AND PRECAUTIONS
May increase sun sensitivity in some individuals. Do not take with prescription antidepressants, or cough syrups containing dextromethorphan, as this can result in a very dangerous interaction known as serotonin syndrome. As this herb has a well-documented impact on the metabolism of certain medication, please discuss Saint John's wort use with your physician or pharmacist. If you are pregnant, nursing or taking prescription medication, please consult your physician before taking this or any other herb.

LOOK-ALIKES: Ragwort (*Jacobaea vulgaris*) TOXIC

IDENTIFY & GROW

🌼 TYPE OF PLANT: Perennial

🌼 HABITAT: Unpicky about soil conditions and moisture, Saint John's wort grows in disturbed areas such as pastures, ditches and other wayside locations in sunny spaces that deliver some protection from scorching afternoon sun.

🌼 HEIGHT: 1–3' (0.6–1 m)

🌼 LEAF: Oblong, opposite leaves that display tiny transparent "dots" (glands) when held up to the light, giving them a "perforated" appearance

🌼 STEM: Single or multi-stemmed with extensive "branching" toward the top of the plant

🌼 FLOWER: Five-petaled, yellow ½–1½" (1.5–4-cm) flowers

🌼 GROWING INFORMATION: Saint John's wort can be propagated by stem cuttings or seed. Soak seeds in warm water for 4 to 12 hours to help ensure a good germinating rate. Seeds can be sown directly in spring or started indoors. Space your plants 12–18" (30–45 cm) apart. Check your county extension office before planting, as it is considered a noxious weed in some areas.

🌼 FORAGE OR GROW? Due to Saint John's wort's potential status as a "noxious weed" in certain locations, special consideration must be given before planting this herb. This is an herb to forage.

BEST HARVEST PRACTICES
FLOWERING TOPS HARVEST WINDOW: Early to mid-summer

Leaves, stems and flowering tops can be harvested through summer into early fall. The ideal time to harvest is just as the first flowers start to open.

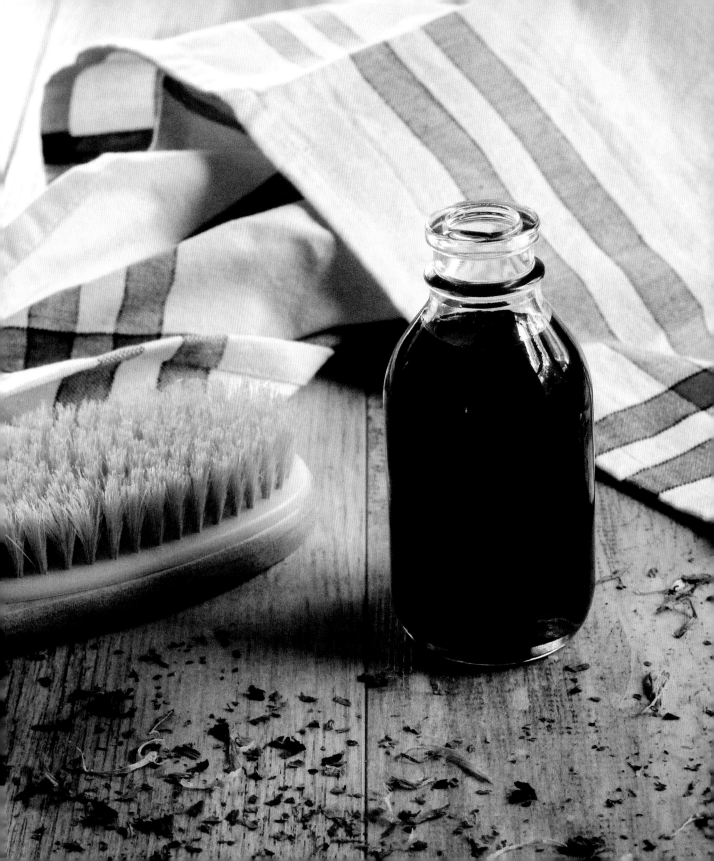

SAINT JOHN'S WORT MASSAGE OIL FOR NERVE PAIN

Saint John's wort is one of the rare herbs that I infuse fresh (well, slightly wilted) into oil. Doing so produces one of the most amazing garnet-hued oils. It is truly a sight to behold. This specialty infusion method helps to drive off excess moisture while also imparting the oil with the rich red medicine of the herb.

In this recipe, I also add lemon balm, making it an excellent remedy for viral nerve pain as observed in shingles. If your nerve pain is not viral in nature, feel free to leave it out.

YIELD: 1 pint (480 ml)

INGREDIENTS

2 cups (480 ml) olive oil

1 cup (50 g) chopped fresh Saint John's wort leaves and flower, wilted for 4–6 hours

¼ cup (6 g) dried lemon balm (optional)

INSTRUCTIONS

To properly infuse fresh Saint John's wort (and lemon balm, if desired) into oil, I use a modified version of the heated oil infusion method detailed on page 12. Instead of placing a lid on the jar, place an upside-down coffee filter or a small washcloth over the top of the jar and rubber band in place. It is also necessary to increase the heat to high when you are near enough to the slow cooker to replace the water as it evaporates; dial the slow cooker down to its lowest setting when unattended. The oil is finished when it has taken on a deep garnet tone. Strain the oil through two layers of flour sack cloth into a liquid measuring cup. Pour into a bottle with a flip top closure to make for ease of use.

Due to the increased chance for spoilage because of the presence of moisture in the herb, get to know the aroma of this oil well to help you detect if it has gone "off." Store in a cool, dry place. Use within 1 year.

Adult use: Massage into affected areas of nerve pain. If your child is experiencing nerve pain or shingles, please consult your physician.

WILD ROSE

OTHER COMMON NAMES: There are thousands of rose types and names

LATIN NAME: *Rosa* sp.

HERBAL ENERGETICS: cool/neutral

THERAPEUTIC ACTIONS: alterative, antibacterial, antidepressant, anti-inflammatory, antioxidant, antiseptic, antispasmodic, antiviral, anxiolytic, aphrodisiac, astringent, cardiovascular, cholagogue, diaphoretic, digestive, diuretic, emmenagogue, expectorant, hypotensive, tonic, vulnerary

PARTS USED: flower, hips (fall fruit)

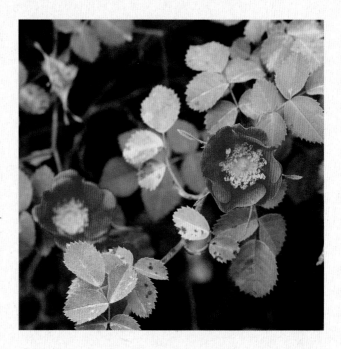

HERBAL MONOGRAPH

Rose is the botanical on which legends are built. Rose allegory and myth first appear in written record as long ago as ancient Mesopotamia, after which the Greeks and Romans wove this most fragrant botanical into many tales. The Greek goddess Chloris declared the rose the undisputed queen of the floral kingdom, and some many years later early Christians dedicated the rose to the Virgin Mary, dubbing her the Rosa mystica. Aesop spins a poetic tale of a meeting of flowers, for which rose arrives too late but being ever-favored the rose could stand alone as queen. From fairy fable to Christianity, the rose is tied to a variety of emotions and virtues. In our modern Western culture, the rose is closely associated with love, as it has been throughout much of written history. Looking deeper we see rose also symbolizing innocence and protection. And there is hardly a botanical that offers a clearer message about boundaries than rose. To gather her beauty (and medicinal benefits), one must be respectful of her thorns.

In the Ayurvedic tradition of medicine, rose is the great balancer. Rose takes excess and moves it to areas of deficiency, particularly when we are speaking of "heat." This is often observed as external heat, such as reddened, marbled, splotchy skin, with signs of visceral cold (like sluggish digestion). I reach for rose when I want to harmonize a formula, as its flavor is calm and inviting and its energetics are gentle. Rose is never an herb with a heavy hand; rather it invites balance and healing.

Rose is closely associated with matters of the heart. Often, we see this botanical being linked to our emotional hearts and rightly so. Rose possesses a euphoric aphrodisiac quality and seems to soften the edges of anxiety and self-doubt. It is naturally uplifting and appears to have a calming effect on blood pressure and speedy pulse. Rose also acts on the cardiovascular system in a more mechanical way in offering excellent vitamin C stores by way of the petals and even more so from the hips.

Not limited to affairs of the heart (metaphorical and physical), rose is often used for digestive and urinary complaints. A gentle tonifying astringent with antispasmodic action, rose firms and supports lax tissue. These properties make this botanical ideally suited to those with upper abdominal cramping, mucus in the digestive system and diarrhea. A simple tea of chamomile flowers and rose petals will soothe any number of digestive complaints and calm nervous dyspepsia.

Rose is also a cardinal herb for female sexual health. As a libido-boosting aphrodisiac, there is little question regarding its ability to put folks in the right frame of mind for romance. Moreover though, it is a nourishing and supportive herb for more intimate concerns such as feminine itching, vaginal dryness, menstrual cramping, excessive bleeding, pelvic congestion and prolapse.

Considering its association with beauty, rose is an unsurprising botanical for the skin. The alluring perfume of rose is simply enough to make one feel beautiful and desired. Beyond its euphoric aroma, rose petals and rose hips are truly indispensable in herbal skin care. Rose petals are exceptionally soothing to hot, dry skin conditions, such as rosacea and sun or windburn, while also promoting firmness. As a humectant, rose actually draws atmospheric moisture to the skin, encouraging a plump, radiant complexion and reducing the appearance of fine lines. Rose hips are an excellent source of vitamin C and can be used to speed the skin's natural renewal process to reveal positively glowing, baby-soft skin and reduce discoloration and scarring.

BEST PREPARATIONS: Rose is a versatile herb with a variety of applications both internal and external. Teas and infusions made from rose petals and rose hips are full of alluring flavor and medicinal benefits. I prefer to prepare tinctures from fresh plant material, but dried herb is also fine to work with. Due to the relatively high moisture content of petals and rose hips, oil infusions should be crafted with dried herb.

Skincare items such as creams and serums can be made with infused oils and aqueous menstruums, such as witch hazel and vegetable glycerin. Fine aromatic hydrosols can be crafted from distillation of the petals. Additionally, rose hips yield an exceptional pressed oil.

Rose petals and rose hips are fascinating and ephemeral flavors when added to jams, jellies and baked goods. Beverages prepared with rose have a hint of the divine.

HERBAL SUBSTITUTES: Calendula (*Calendula officinalis*): vulnerary | Lavender (*Lavandula angustifolia*): sedative

SAFETY AND PRECAUTIONS
Rose is widely considered safe. If you are pregnant, nursing or taking prescription medication, please consult you physician before taking this or any other herb.

LOOK-ALIKES: Other cultivated *Rosa* species

IDENTIFY & GROW

🌸 **TYPE OF PLANT:** Perennial

🌸 **HABITAT:** Roses prefer full sun, rich soils and adequate moisture. Wild roses are often observed along roadsides, property lines and near waterways and ditches.

🌸 **HEIGHT:** A somewhat sprawling habit with arching canes reaching 3–15' (1–5 m)

🌸 **LEAF:** Alternate leaves with 5 to 9 serrated leaflets; green with new growth sometimes blushing bronze-red

🌸 **STEM:** Prominent prickly thorns

🌸 **FLOWER:** White to pink five-petaled flowers with prominent yellow stamens in the center appear late spring into early summer

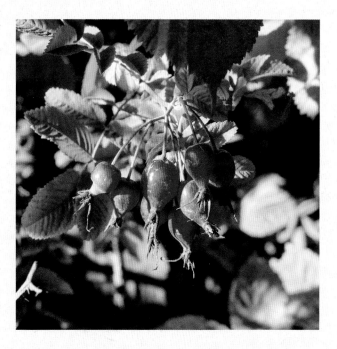

🌸 **FRUIT:** Flowers mature into red ovoid to round fruits in early to late fall

🌸 **GROWING INFORMATION:** Roses are most easily propagated by division. Dig suckers in early spring or fall and transplant to a sunny location with fertile soils. Trim to about 6" (15 cm) above ground level to promote good root system development.

🌸 **FORAGE OR GROW?** Wild roses may be a bit unruly for a suburban landscape, making this botanical a good one for most foragers. Cultivated and hybrid tea varieties of rose are suitable for any landscape, but have a somewhat reduced medicinal value and rarely produce adequate hips.

BEST HARVEST PRACTICES
FLOWER HARVEST WINDOW: Late spring

HIP (BERRY) HARVEST WINDOW: Fall

Wild rose is easily identified. Gather petals in spring, leaving the stamens intact to develop a hip. Harvest red rose hips after the first frost to encourage flavor and sweetness.

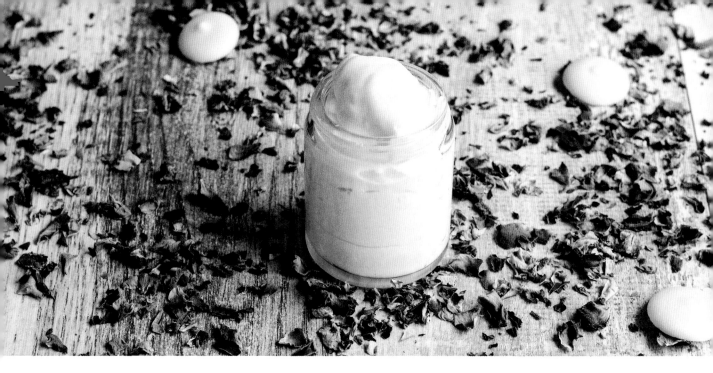

FIRMING WILD ROSE UNDEREYE CREAM

Roses are luxurious. So are eye creams. Can you imagine a more luxurious treat for the delicate skin around your eyes?

This heavenly formula is an absolute olfactory treat, and it's an incredibly rich and nourishing cream for the skin around the eyes. This cream promotes firm, soft skin and reduces the appearance of fine lines and puffiness. Since this cream is not chemically preserved, it must be refrigerated between uses and discarded after 2 weeks.

YIELD: 2 ounces (60 ml)

INGREDIENTS

1 tbsp (15 g) coconut oil or oil of your choice

1 tbsp (15 g) cocoa butter

1 tbsp (1 g) dried wild rose petals

1 tbsp (12 g) emulsifying wax pastilles

1 tbsp (15 ml) rose hip seed oil

3–5 tbsp (45–75 ml) rose water or distilled water

INSTRUCTIONS

Using the double boiler method, infuse the coconut oil and cocoa butter with the rose petals. Strain the infused oil through a fine-mesh sieve and return to the double boiler. Add the emulsifying wax and rose hip seed oil, and heat just until the wax is melted. Remove from the heat, and set aside. Meanwhile, gently raise the temperature of the rose water to within about 10 degrees of the oils. In a small blender or with a handheld beater, slowly pour the rose water into the oils to emulsify. Spoon or pipe into a 2-ounce (60-ml) container.

Apply using your ring fingers, taking special care not to tug at the delicate skin around the eyes. Refrigerate between uses. Use within 2 weeks.

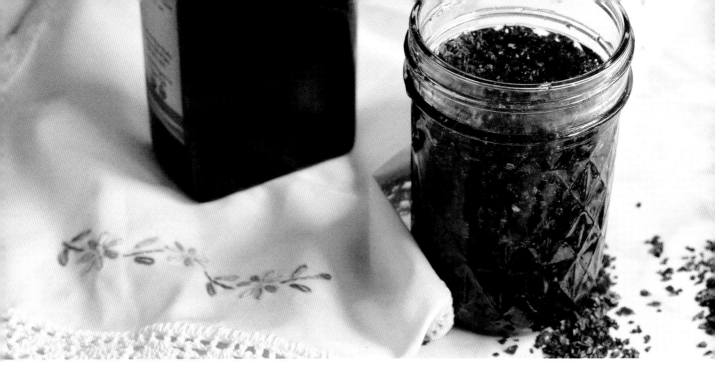

SKIN BRIGHTENING ROSE HIP SERUM

Rose hips pack a mega dose of vitamin C, which provides remarkable benefits for the skin. This serum will help to brighten your complexion and promote radiant, smooth skin. Use this serum along with your regular moisturizer at night. Consider a hat or some UV protection during the day (such as the self heal antioxidant oil on page 43) during the day, especially when exposed to the sun.

Vegetable glycerin fills the multiple roles in this blend. It extracts the amazing rose hip constituents, while also serving as a preservative and acting as a humectant to draw moisture to the skin. Aloe vera gel is also deeply nourishing, fights redness and encourages a hydrated complexion.

YIELD: 4 ounces (120 ml)

INGREDIENTS

¼ cup (35 g) fresh rose hips, chopped (use ¼ cup [25 g] if dried)

½ cup (120 ml) vegetable glycerin

½ cup (120 ml) aloe vera gel

INSTRUCTIONS

Using the regular infusion method (page 12), infuse the rose hips in the glycerin for a minimum of 6 weeks. After the infusion is complete, strain through a fine-mesh sieve into a liquid measuring cup. Add the aloe vera gel, and mix well. Pour into 1- or 2-ounce (30- or 60-ml) amber glass dropper bottles.

To apply, warm 1 or 2 droppers full (1.5 or 3 ml) in between your palms. Press onto your clean, dry face, neck and chest, avoiding the eye area. Follow with your nightly moisturizer. Use within 1 year.

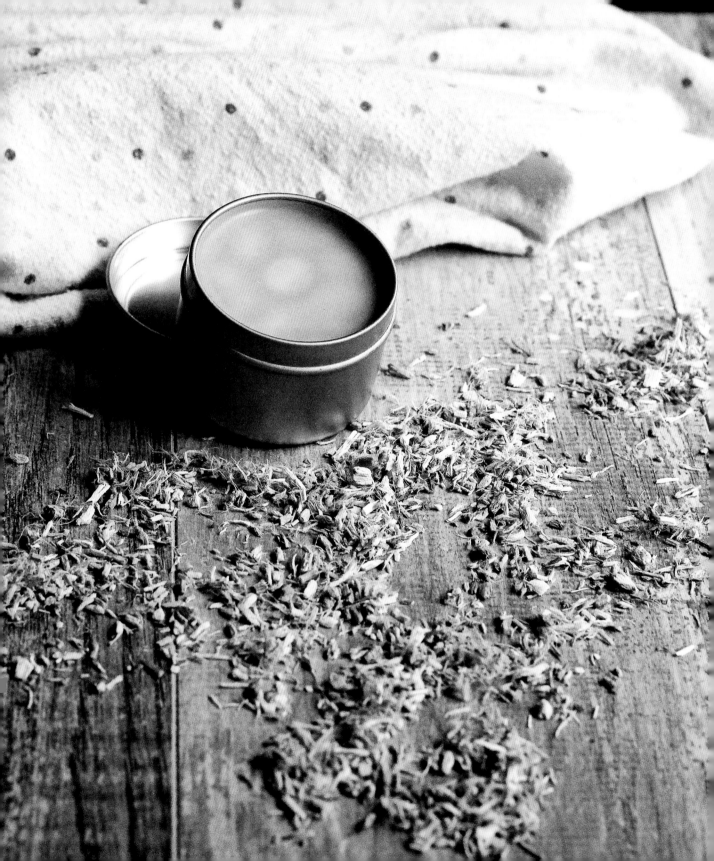

MARSHLAND AND WATERSIDE WONDERS FOR HOLISTIC HEALTH

THERE IS NARY A MORE RESTFUL SOUND than water rushing through rocks and reeds or burbling up in a spring. These waterside habitats are teaming with beauty, but more importantly, with resilience. For every calm creek-side moment there was once a torrent of rushing storm waters in the same place. Waterside medicine is teaching us of perseverance and staying firmly rooted.

Nourishing, immune- and adrenal-supporting green nettle teaches us to always be careful and mindful as we wander our path. Towering, graceful spires of black cohosh, known for its ability to relieve menopausal complaint and support the flexibility of the spinal column, show us how to bend and arch to pressure but not break. Even tender little diuretic cleavers demonstrate how to climb and adapt while shedding unneeded weight. These waterside botanicals show us the magic in ourselves.

STINGING NETTLE

OTHER COMMON NAMES: common nettle, nettle

LATIN NAME: *Urtica dioica, U. urens, U. membranacea*

HERBAL ENERGETICS: cool /dry

THERAPEUTIC ACTIONS: alterative, anodyne, anthelmintic, antiallergenic, antihistamine, anti-inflammatory, anti-rheumatic, astringent, decongestant, diuretic, expectorant, galactagogue, hypoglycemic, nephritic, nutritive, rubefacient, stimulant, tonic

PARTS USED: leaf, seed, root

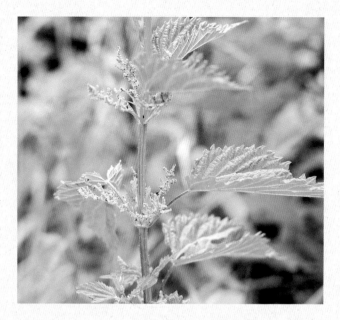

HERBAL MONOGRAPH

It is unlikely that you will ever forget your first (accidental) encounter with stinging nettle. Somehow, I made it well into adulthood before I fully understood the gravity of its moniker. Thrusting my bare arm up to the shoulder into a weedy, overgrown border to gather up a wandering hen, I was shocked by the burning "pins and needles" sensation that ensconced my arm. My husband quickly grabbed some nearby sword fern (one of a few forest-y antidotes to the bite of nettle) and vigorously rubbed my arm, dialing down the pain from searing to simmering. So, this is the "stinging" that we always avoid on our hikes through the woods, I thought. Despite its nasty defenses—harmless save the infuriating irritation—it is a kingly herb worthy of the trouble it takes to gather. Stinging nettle is a botanical that this herbalist would never do without.

Stinging nettle is an herb with a multitude of therapeutic actions and medicinal uses. Its benefits are not limited to a solitary ailment or organ system. Instead, nettle acts on the whole body with virtually unparalleled nutrition—tonifying organs and boosting the actions of many organ systems. Nettle is widely considered to be one of the most mineral-rich, nutritious plant foods, containing significant amounts of calcium, iron, magnesium, zinc, potassium, phosphorous and sodium. Courtesy of its stinging barbs, nettle is also a valuable source of silica. Additionally, this botanical contains vitamins A, C, K and many B vitamins as well as a rich amino acid profile. Stinging nettle infusions and foodstuffs are an excellent source of nutrition for the weak and feeble, those recovering from illness, as well as nursing mothers so long as no contraindications exist. A small recent study demonstrated that nettle tea contributed to increased milk production in the mothers of preterm babies by a statistically significant 80 percent in a seven-day period, with the placebo group only observing a 30 percent increase in breast milk production.

Perhaps one of the most profound uses for stinging nettle is its antiallergenic/antihistamine action. Herbalists have long used this herb to combat seasonal allergies, hay fever and other allergenic conditions. A number of preliminary studies indicate that allergy sufferers are finding as great or greater relief from seasonal allergy symptoms using nettle products than common over-the-counter and prescription allergy medications. Beyond symptoms of sneezy noses and itchy, watery eyes, my own experience and that of several of my clients is that nettle also assists those with high histamine levels due to stress and poor adrenal function manifesting in irritated itchy skin, especially about the face and neck, when upset or under duress. For all heightened allergenic responses, nettle is ideally taken long term—and, in the case of seasonal allergies, at least two months before the peak season of the offending botanical. An interesting study of prolonged induced stress on the mouse model showed that mice receiving nettle leaf extract demonstrated a far greater ability to adapt to stress with improved cognition, muscle coordination and reduced anxiety compared to the untreated control group.

Nettle has a long-standing reputation for its pain-relieving benefits with osteo- and rheumatoid arthritis sufferers. In what may seem to some as highly counterintuitive, it is actually the barbed underside of the leaf that is applied to the skin of the affected areas that appears to bring fairly lasting relief to arthritic pain. This widespread folk treatment is notably not for the faint of heart.

This powerful herb is also known for its profound benefits on the urinary tract system as well as having many other applications. As a diuretic, stinging nettle helps to decrease retaining water, reduce stone size and flush uric acid from the system, making this herb ideal for urinary tract infections, mild kidney stones and gout. The leaf and root are wonderfully astringent, making a nettle decoction an effective and nutritive remedy for diarrhea complaints. As a styptic/hemostatic herb, nettle is also associated with reducing blood loss. It is a common ingredient in herbal hair loss remedies due to its tonifying and stimulating effects on the scalp. Additionally, nettle has been shown to help stabilize blood glucose levels.

BEST PREPARATIONS: Nettle is a very versatile herb. The fresh leaves are often used for culinary purposes, making a delicious substitute for spinach or kale in cooked recipes. Cooking neutralizes the sting. Fresh leaves can also be blended into an amazing, nutritious pesto or even a green smoothie— also free of the pesky sting. Late-season seeds are a wonderful addition to seasoning blends.

Nettle leaves are the most commonly used part. They can be dried and stored in a cool, dry place for use in teas and infusions. They can also be tinctured either fresh or dry, using alcohol or vinegar as the menstruum. Roots are less commonly used, but they should be dried and used for long simmering decoctions. Although seldom used as a medicinal preparation, nettle seeds can be used ground to a powder and encapsulated, or simply eaten.

As nettle is a somewhat drying and astringent herb, use thoughtfully when combining with herbs possessing similar action, such as yellow dock and Oregon grape root. Due to its high iron content, nettle combines well with herbs high in vitamin C such as rose hips and pine needles. Members of the mint family also make for flavorful and cooling teas that often assist with the inflammation associated with seasonal allergies.

SAFETY AND PRECAUTIONS
Stinging nettle is widely regarded as safe. Due to its stimulating and diuretic effects, nettle should not be used by women in the early stages of pregnancy and those with kidney disease. Those taking medication for diabetes, high blood pressure or bleeding/clotting issues should avoid nettle until they consult with a health professional.

LOOK-ALIKES: Wood nettle (*Laportea canadensis*)

IDENTIFY & GROW
TYPE OF PLANT: Perennial

HABITAT: Nettle is a common understory plant, growing in moist, relatively pH neutral soils in shady woodland areas, along streams and open ditches. Habitats can be found from sea level to sub-alpine elevations.

HEIGHT: 4–6' (1–2 m)

LEAF: Finely serrated (toothed), somewhat heart-shaped leaves ranging from vibrant green to a bronze-purple in color. Leaf undersides are covered in tiny silica barbs; the topside is barb free.

STEM: The fibrous stem is covered with stinging barbs up the length of the stem, with leaves arranged opposite one another. Plants can regularly reach heights of 4–6' (1–2 m), but have been known to grow even taller under ideal conditions.

FLOWER: Small, unassuming greenish-white inflorescence (catkin-like) appearing early to mid-summer atop

SEED: Seed inflorescence appears late summer to early fall following flowering.

GROWING INFORMATION: Nettle seeds can be started indoors 4 to 6 weeks before the last frost in your area. Nettle seeds should be placed in a peat-rich starting medium and kept evenly moist. Germination is expected in about 14 days. Nettle seeds can also be directly sown. Transplants or directly sown seed should be planted in moist rich soil with partial or dappled shade. You should also take care to plant stinging nettle where stinging contact can be avoided, such as the back of a shady border or in an open wooded area.

FORAGE OR GROW? Nettle might be a bit unfriendly with its prickly defenses for the average home garden, so my vote is that this is a botanical to forage.

BEST HARVEST PRACTICES
LEAF HARVEST WINDOW: Early spring through early summer

SEED HARVEST WINDOW: Mid-summer

Nettle leaves can be harvested by pinching the upper side of the leaf to pluck without sting, although this is somewhat tedious. New growth will be the tenderest for edible purposes, but all leaves can be harvested and processed for medicinal purposes. Seeds can be harvested at maturity. It is recommended to wear sturdy gloves and long sleeves when harvesting.

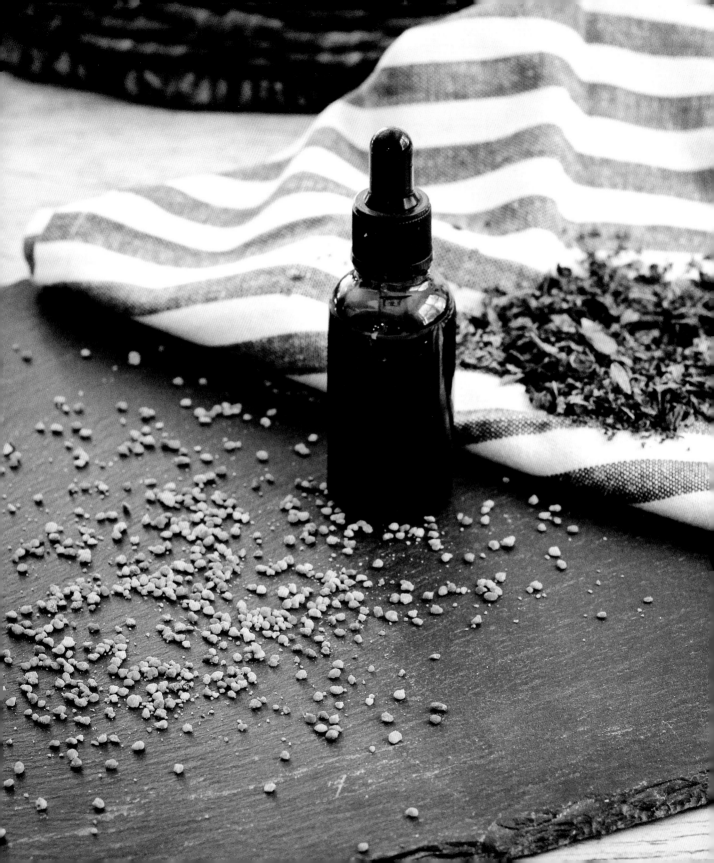

ALLERGY SEASON SAVIOR TINCTURE

Considering the long-term medicinal benefits of nettle, I like to make enough of this tincture to last all year and well into the next—just to be safe and never run out before the next batch is ready. This is to say that this is a tincture I would never be without in my home apothecary.

Nettle provides excellent histamine relief and allergenic response support. The addition of bee pollen adds B vitamins and quercetin. This tincture is equally appropriate for those with seasonal allergy symptoms or elevated histamine levels due to adrenal fatigue/dysfunction.

YIELD: 1 quart (approximately 1 L)

ADULT DOSE: 2–3 droppers full (3–4.5 ml), 3 times daily

CHILD'S DOSE, AGES 6–12: 1–2 droppers full (1.5–3 ml), 3 times daily

CHILD'S DOSE, AGES 2–6: 5–15 drops, 3 times daily

INGREDIENTS

32 oz (950 ml) 100 proof vodka

6½ oz (185 g) fresh nettle leaves, chopped

3 oz (85 g) bee pollen granules

INSTRUCTIONS

Combine all the ingredients in a jar with a tight-fitting lid, large enough to accommodate the contents. Infuse the vodka with the nettle and bee pollen for at least 6 weeks. After the infusion is complete, strain the tincture through two layers of cheese cloth or muslin, squeezing to remove as much liquid as possible. Discard the spent marc in the compost, and bottle the tincture in an amber glass master bottle or individual 1- or 2-ounce (30- or 60-ml) bottles. Use within 1 year.

NETTLE & PEPPERMINT NOURISHING HERBAL INFUSION FOR ALLERGY SEASON

This super refreshing blend of peppermint and nettle offers cooling soothing relief during allergy attacks. The calming and cooling effects of the mint combined with the antihistamine action of nettle is sure to ameliorate the itching, sneezing nose and the watering eyes. Drink this as an iced nourishing herbal infusion to really take advantage of its "coolness."

YIELD: 4 cups (100 g) of blend

ADULT DOSE: 16–32 ounces (480–960 ml) sipped throughout the day

CHILD'S DOSE, AGES 6–12: 8 ounces (240 ml) once a day

INGREDIENTS

2 cups (50 g) dried nettle leaf

2 cups (50 g) dried peppermint

INSTRUCTIONS

Combine the herbs, and store in a tight-lidded jar in a cool, dry place.

To prepare the infusion: Add 2 to 3 tablespoons (3 to 5 g) of the herbal blend to a quart-sized (1-L) jar. Fill the jar with water just off the boil. Allow the jar to cool for at least 30 minutes, then move the jar to the refrigerator to cool, and infuse for 6 to 12 hours. After infusing, strain the infusion and pour over ice. Store unused infusion in the refrigerator. Use the dried blend within 1 year.

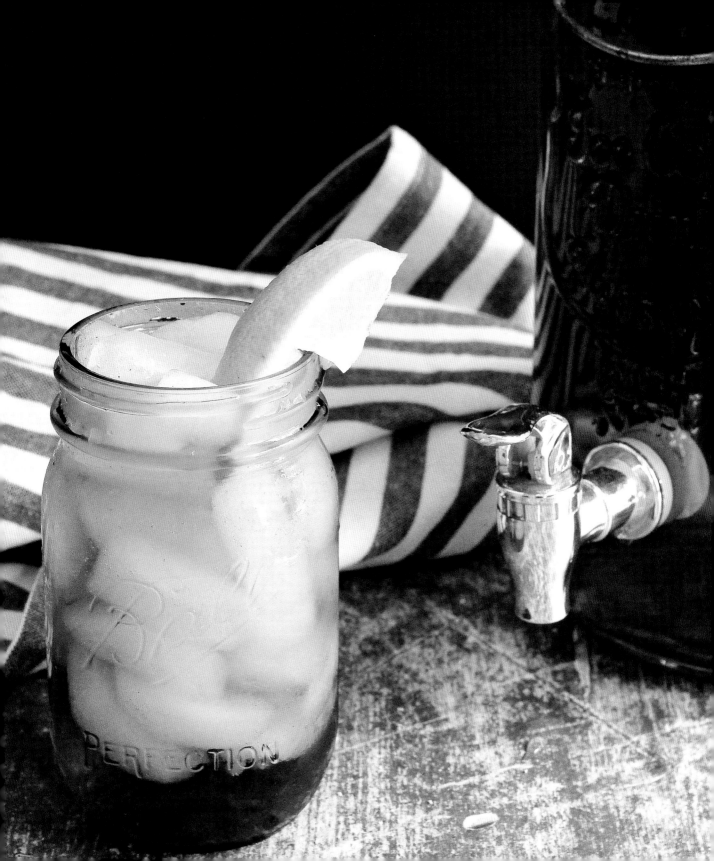

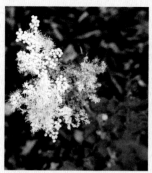
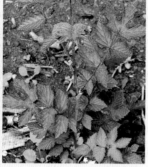

MEADOWSWEET

OTHER COMMON NAMES: bridewort, Quaker lady, Queen of the Meadow

LATIN NAME: *Filipendula ulmaria*

HERBAL ENERGETICS: cool/dry

THERAPEUTIC ACTIONS: alterative, analgesic, antacid, antiemetic, anti-inflammatory, antimicrobial, anti-rheumatic, antiseptic, cardiovascular, carminative, diaphoretic, digestive, diuretic, febrifuge, tonic

PARTS USED: leaf, flower

HERBAL MONOGRAPH

Some herbs are considered sacred to certain cultures and religions. Meadowsweet was to the ancient Druids, and it is not hard to understand why. Meadowsweet is perfection in plant form. Wild yet stately, and very medicinally valuable.

Meadowsweet is a much-heralded herb for the digestive system. More directly, it is one of the only herbs indicated for acute ulcer complaints. Meadowsweet's unique medicinal actions combine pain relief with the promotion of the secretion of gastric juices. It protects the stomach lining from the effects of hyperacidity, neutralizing many complaints before they even start and healing those that currently exist. Meadowsweet is suited for the individual plagued by acid reflux and heartburn, sour stomach, acidic breath and metallic taste in the mouth.

Meadowsweet owes its pain-relieving action to a constituent called salicylaldehyde, the active constituent of aspirin. As such, meadowsweet offers relief to those with stiff, painful joints, headaches (including migraines) and hot, red-faced fevers. Much like aspirin, it is not an appropriate herb to use with small children with a fever for the increased risk of Reye's syndrome. Its diuretic properties make it an excellent herb for those with gout and rheumatoid arthritis and for those with urinary tract complaints such as retained urine, cystitis and weak pelvic floor.

Topically, meadowsweet offers gentle astringent action combined with anti-inflammatory properties. This makes it an ideal herb for those with puffy eyes, and is also helpful for persistent redness and heat in the complexion such as that observed in rosacea. Cooled infusions of meadowsweet applied to teary or allergic eyes or reddened inflamed skin can bring cool, calming relief to these areas.

BEST PREPARATIONS: Meadowsweet makes for bittersweet and slightly aromatic teas and infusions. The herb should be tinctured when fresh. Witch hazel extract can be infused with the herb for a soothing facial mist. It is also a lovely ingredient in homemade mead!

HERBAL SUBSTITUTES: Cottonwood (*Populus trichocarpa*): analgesic | marshmallow (*Althea officinalis*): heartburn

SAFETY AND PRECAUTIONS

Do not use if you have an aspirin allergy or with children with fevers. If you are pregnant, nursing or taking prescription medication, please consult your physician before using this or any other herb.

LOOK-ALIKES: Astilbe (*Astilbe* sp.)

IDENTIFY & GROW

TYPE OF PLANT: Perennial

HABITAT: Meadowsweet likes the dappled shade of the forest edge and deep, moist soil. Native to Europe but tends to naturalize in hospitable conditions.

HEIGHT: 3–6' (1–2 m)

LEAF: Dark, deeply veined, pinnate leaves with a lighter, somewhat downy underside

FLOWER: Frothy, white or sometimes pink-purple, clusters of tiny flowers; appear June through September emitting a heady, sweet vanilla-almond-honey fragrance

GROWING INFORMATION: Meadowsweet seeds can be sown in fall or planted in spring after cold stratification. Plant in partial shade, in an area with ample moisture, but not boggy conditions. May require staking in shadier location. Divide every 3 years to avoid overcrowding.

FORAGE OR GROW? In many areas of its native Europe, meadowsweet is easily identified and foraged. In North America, this herb is best to grow.

BEST HARVEST PRACTICES

LEAF & FLOWER HARVEST WINDOW: Mid-summer Harvest leaves and flower when plant is in bloom. Tincture immediately or dry quickly.

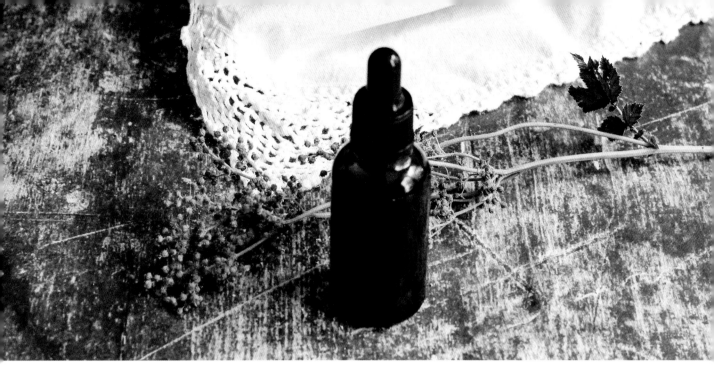

 ## MEADOWSWEET BITTERS FOR HEARTBURN & REFLUX

Meadowsweet is a gorgeous herb with the most intoxicating aroma. It would only stand to reason that this magical plant works magic on our insides. As one of the most effective herbal remedies against heartburn and acid reflux, this tincture helps to make mealtime less worrisome. This tincture is also an effective pain reliever, but should be not be administered to children with a fever due to increased risk of Reye's syndrome.

YIELD: 1 pint (480 ml)

ADULT DOSE: 1–2½ droppers full (1.5–4 ml), 3 times daily

NOT RECOMMENDED FOR CHILDREN.
If your child is experiencing frequent heartburn or reflux, please consult your physician.

INGREDIENTS

2 cups (480 ml) 100 proof spirits

1½ cups (65 g) fresh meadowsweet leaf and flower, chopped finely

INSTRUCTIONS

Combine the spirits and meadowsweet in a jar with a tight-fitting lid. Infuse for a minimum of 6 weeks, shaking daily. When the infusion is complete, strain through two layers of flour sack cloth into a liquid measuring cup. Pour into 1- or 2-ounce (30- or 60-ml) amber glass dropper bottles or into a pint-sized (480-ml) amber glass master bottle for dispensing. Use within 1 year.

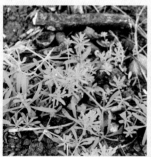
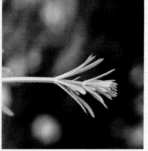

CLEAVERS

OTHER COMMON NAMES: bedstraw, catchweed, goosegrass, clivers

LATIN NAME: *Galium aparine*

HERBAL ENERGETICS: cool/dry

THERAPEUTIC ACTIONS: alterative, antiarthritic, anti-inflammatory, astringent, cardiovascular, diaphoretic, diuretic, lymphatic, tonic, vulnerary

PARTS USED: aboveground parts

HERBAL MONOGRAPH

Cleavers is an herb that always brings a smile to my face. It happily grows in damp and shady spots and is easy to identify. And it is often very, very prolific.

Perhaps a nod to its damp, cool habitat, this clingy weed is an herb that simply knows what to do with excess water. Cleavers has very specific applications to water retention and edema and is ideally suited to those with a boggy sensation in the bladder (suggestive of retained urine), incontinence (including bedwetting in preschool and school-age children) and inflammation of the urethra. Cleavers has also been shown to have a normalizing effect on blood pressure and a reduction in arthritic, gout and kidney complaints. Cleavers may also help with concerns of an enlarged prostate and poor urinary pressure in men.

Cleavers is also known for its great affinity for the lymphatic system. This herb is ideal for complaints of "sluggish lymph," and more acutely for instances of lymphedema. It is also used to address hardened and swollen nodes around the neck and armpit, as well as to reduce sebaceous cysts near the neck and jawline. Externally it is used to calm and cool inflammatory conditions of the skin, such as eczema, psoriasis, acne and painful bug bites and stings.

BEST PREPARATIONS: Cleavers is an herb that is ideally used in its fresh form—either prepared as a tincture, an expressed juice known as a succus, or applied externally as a poultice. Some herbalists use the dry herb as a cold infusion to harness the full range of its constituents. As cleavers is in the same general plant family as coffee, the dried herb seeds can be lightly roasted and used as a coffee substitute.

HERBAL SUBSTITUTES: uva-ursi (*Arctostaphylos uva-ursi*): urinary complaints | burdock (*Articum lappa*): skin concerns

SAFETY AND PRECAUTIONS

Cleavers are generally considered safe, but should be avoided by those with kidney disease. If you are pregnant, nursing or taking prescription medication, please consult your physician before using this or any other herb.

LOOK-ALIKES: Sweet woodruff (*Galium odoratum*)

IDENTIFY & GROW

TYPE OF PLANT: Annual

HABITAT: Cleavers are often observed in dense to part shade, and are frequently found under deciduous trees that drop copious leaves in fall, providing a moisture-retentive mulch. Cleavers creep along the ground or grow up sturdier plant material.

HEIGHT: Cleavers spread horizontally unless "climbing" on other plant material. Stems can reach from 1–3 feet (0.3–1 m) in length.

LEAF: Simple narrow lance-oval leaves arranged in whorls of 6 to 8; tiny barb-shaped hairs give the plant a "sticky" feel

STEM: Angular or square with many minute "sticky" hairs

FLOWER: Small white to greenish star-shaped flowers appearing spring to early summer

SEED: "Fuzzy" burr-like seeds

GROWING INFORMATION: Cleavers seeds should be sown in the fall, directly into beds with plenty of organic matter such as leaf litter. Once established, cleavers reseeds itself readily.

FORAGE OR GROW? While one could certainly grow cleavers, it might be considered slightly unsightly to less appreciative neighbors. Due to its ease of identification and prolific nature, cleavers is an herb to forage.

BEST HARVEST PRACTICES
ABOVEGROUND PARTS HARVEST WINDOW: Spring

Harvest all aboveground parts during late spring and early summer just as the flowers begin to bloom. Chop finely for immediate tincturing or dry quickly without the use of high heat, which may damage its constituents.

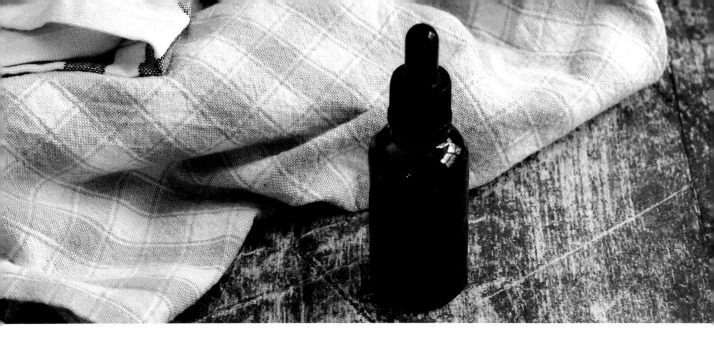

CLEAVERS TINCTURE WITH DANDELION FOR WATER RETENTION

Retained water doesn't sound all that "bad," but for those of you who deal with this very common issue, you know just how frustrating it can be. From tender midsection, uncomfortable waist lines, puffy eyes and spongy joints—retained water is not just a nuisance, but can have long-term health implications such as high blood pressure.

Many people are retaining water without knowing it. Your wedding ring is suddenly uncomfortably tight—that's probably retained water. Pillowy undereye area—retained water. Pants that fit some days but not others—retained water, I tell you. Rid yourself of excess fluid with the combined gentle action of cleavers and dandelion leaf. Both cleavers and dandelion make their appearance in early spring and can be found in many climates.

YIELD: 1 pint (480 ml)

ADULT DOSE: 2–5 droppers (3–7.5 ml), 3 times daily

NOT RECOMMENDED FOR CHILDREN.
If your child is showing signs of fluid retention, please consult your physician.

INGREDIENTS

2 cups (480 ml) 80 proof spirits (vodka recommended)

¾ cup (40 g) chopped fresh cleavers

¼ cup (15 g) chopped fresh dandelion greens

INSTRUCTIONS

Place the spirits, cleavers and dandelion in a jar with a tight-fitting lid. Infuse the spirits with the herbs for a minimum of 6 weeks, shaking daily. After the infusion is complete, strain through two layers of flour sack cloth into a liquid measuring cup, wringing to release all the liquids. Pour the finished tincture into individual 1- or 2-ounce (30- or 60-ml) amber glass dropper bottles or into a pint-sized (480 ml) amber glass master bottle for dispensing. Use within 1 year.

BLACK COHOSH

OTHER COMMON NAMES: bugbane, fairy candle, snakeroot, squawroot

LATIN NAME: *Actaea racemosa* (formerly *Cimicifuga racemosa*)

HERBAL ENERGETICS: cool/dry

THERAPEUTIC ACTIONS: alterative, analgesic, anti-inflammatory, anti-rheumatic, antispasmodic, diaphoretic, emmenagogue, nervine, sedative

PARTS USED: root

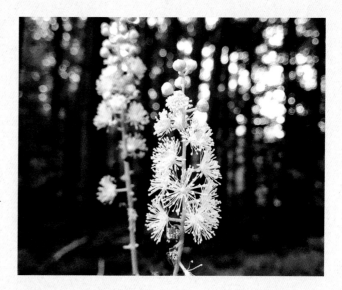

HERBAL MONOGRAPH

Some herbs become so entwined with a condition that we almost forget what else they offer. We see Saint John's wort pigeonholed for depression, lavender for anxiety and we see black cohosh for menopause. While there is little doubt in my herbalist mind that black cohosh is an exceptional herb for menopausal complaints, it is an herb for so much more. Black cohosh is an herb that can teach us about how to find peace in our bodies through pain and shifting hormones. Watching the tall elegant spires of black cohosh sway in a breeze, this herb teaches us how to gracefully yield to pressure yet not be toppled over by it—because our roots are deep and strong. It is an herb about flexibility, bending and releasing so that we can remain strong in our footing.

To say that black cohosh is a "menopausal" herb is incredibly myopic. It doesn't cure menopause. Menopause is not a disease and does not need curing. Rather, black cohosh is an herb that supports a woman's reproductive health in various stages from her first bleed to her last and beyond. Black cohosh offers many of its benefits by stimulating pelvic blood flow and relieving tension and stagnation. Thus, it is very effective for bringing on a delayed or scanty menses and for easing menstrual cramps, especially those that radiate into the upper thigh and pelvis. It can also help ameliorate any sense of fullness and bloating about the pelvic region. It is indicated for uterine cysts and fibroids, heavy menstrual bleeding (often accompanied by diarrhea) and cervical spasm. Midwives use black cohosh as a low dose or as a homeopathic to stimulate weak and irregular contractions into full labor. It is a particularly good herb to address some psychological issues associated with PMS and menopause, such

as brooding, withdrawn behavior, irritability and frustration. Black cohosh helps to promote a good estrogen balance during menopause, and as a cooling sedative, helps to relieve hot flashes and insomnia.

Black cohosh is quite undervalued when it comes to more psychological complaints. It is an herb that helps to address feelings of nervousness and tension. It is the cardinal herb for those that tend to withdraw under times of grief and stress, who struggle to find words to express their pain and appear irritable and dismissive to others. Internally these people often feel apathetic following traumatic experiences. Much like we see black cohosh stimulating the reproductive organs, so too we see it releasing stagnant emotions.

Black cohosh is also an unsung hero(ine) when it comes to pain management. This botanical is indicated for rheumatoid arthritis, sciatica, osteoarthritis, intercostal myalgia (rib pain), muscle spasms and excessive cerebrospinal fluid which can contribute to headache. In a nod to the doctrine of signatures, the tall, graceful, arching black cohosh is used for whiplash injuries with pain in the shoulders, upper back and neck, as well as for ligament and tendon injuries.

Additionally, black cohosh foliage emits a fragrance that deters insects, making it a candidate for an all-natural bug repellant.

BEST PREPARATIONS: Black cohosh should be tinctured fresh.

HERBAL SUBSTITUTES: Red clover (*Trifoium pratense*): hot flashes | shatavari (*Asparagus racemosus*): hormonal regulation

SAFETY AND PRECAUTIONS
Avoid if pregnant or nursing unless under the care of an experienced herbalist or midwife. High doses of this herb can be dangerous.

LOOK-ALIKES: Goat's beard (*Aruncus dioicus*), astilbe (*Astilbe biternate*)

IDENTIFY & GROW
- **TYPE OF PLANT:** Perennial

- **HABITAT:** Black cohosh prefers the dappled shade of wooded meadows and the edges of moist forests.

- **HEIGHT:** 4–8' (1–2.5 m)

- **LEAF:** Deep green leaves are pinnate and compound with serrated margins.

- **STEM:** Tall, sometimes arching stem

- **FLOWER:** Elegant tall spires of tiny white star-like flowers

- **ROOT:** Dark, thick root surrounded by many fibrous rootlets

- **GROWING INFORMATION:** For best germination, black cohosh seeds should be cold stratified before sown in spring. A well-established plant of three years or more can be divided in early spring, or late fall.

- **FORAGE OR GROW?** I vote, unequivocally, that black cohosh is an herb to grow. It is considered an at-risk plant in its native habitat (southeastern North America), and it is a stunning botanical for the shady landscape, adding an interesting vertical element to the garden.

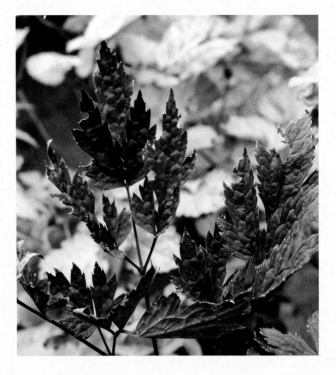

BEST HARVEST PRACTICES
ROOT HARVEST WINDOW: Fall

Dig and divide plants of at least 3 years of age in fall, replanting at least half of the roots for future crops.

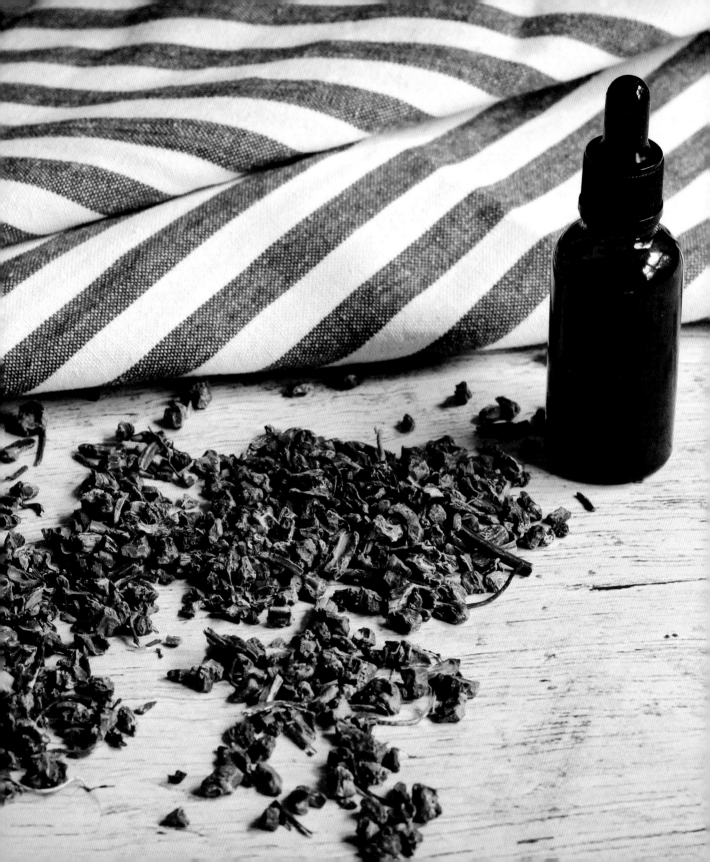

MENOPAUSE MANAGEMENT TINCTURE

While I try not to pigeonhole herbs, there is no denying the fact that black cohosh offers relief to many of the more distressing complaints sometimes associated with menopause. I want to make it emphatically clear: menopause is not a disease, and women experiencing menopause are not in need of fixing. During these times of transition in our biology, we can become imbalanced.

In this tincture, black cohosh coaxes the body back into balance, relieving complaints such as insomnia, irritability and hot flashes. Shatavari root is added to improve libido and vaginal tone, while also decreasing vaginal dryness.

YIELD: 1 pint (480 ml)

ADULT DOSE: About 1⅓ droppers full (2 ml), 3 times daily

INGREDIENTS

2 cups (480 ml) 100 proof spirits (vodka recommended)

1 cup (125 g) fresh black cohosh root

½ cup (35 g) dried shatavari root

INSTRUCTIONS

Place the spirits, black cohosh root and shatavari root in a jar with a tight-fitting lid. Infuse the spirits with the roots for a minimum of 6 weeks, shaking daily.

When the tincture is adequately infused, strain it through two layers of flour sack cloth or multiple layers of cheese cloth. Wring the cloth to extract as much liquid as possible. Pour strained tincture into 1- or 2-ounce (30- or 60-ml) amber glass dropper bottles, or into a larger amber glass master bottle for dispensing. Use within 1 year.

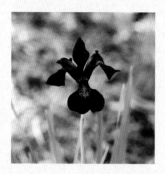

BLUE FLAG IRIS

OTHER COMMON NAMES: poison flag, wild iris, Fleur de Lis, liver lily

LATIN NAME: *Iris versicolor*

HERBAL ENERGETICS: warm/dry. There is some disagreement about iris temperature. I lean toward warm, as it is acidic and acids are traditionally warming.

THERAPEUTIC ACTIONS: alterative, anti-acnegenic, anti-inflammatory, astringent, cholagogue, diaphoretic, diuretic, emetic, hepatic, laxative, lymphatic, pancreatic, purgative, stimulant

PARTS USED: root

HERBAL MONOGRAPH

I had a great internal debate about including this beautiful botanical in my book. It is, after all, a very strong herb with the capability to do harm if misused. But, if used appropriately, it can be an incredibly useful herb in the home apothecary. Ultimately, blue flag iris made the cut.

I will skip directly to why I chose to include blue flag iris. It is a plant that I learned about many years ago while working in the cosmetic and skincare industry. Blue flag iris was used in formulation specific for dehydrated, rough, acne-prone skin. Used externally blue flag iris addresses rough, scaly conditions of the skin as well as cystic acne, especially that which occurs in lymphatic areas such as the jawline. Its acidic properties help to smooth inflamed skin with uneven texture while dissolving sebaceous cysts. This is not an herb for those with oily skin; rather it is better suited for those with surface dryness and hormonal acne. Used properly, blue flag iris promotes a clear and radiant complexion.

When we turn our attention toward internal use of blue flag iris, we must weigh the potential benefit against the potential for side effects. Let it first be mentioned that I would never recommend the use of fresh or raw iris root. Secondly, even use of the dried root should be done only under the supervision of an experienced herbal practitioner. Blue flag iris is considered cathartic, emetic, and purgative—meaning that it can cause violent cramping, vomiting and diarrhea if used inappropriately. However, it has been used historically for those suffering from liver deficiency, poor gall bladder function and extreme constipation. It does so by being extremely stimulating to the digestive organs and the bowels, and therefore can be a difficult herb to moderate in its action.

BEST PREPARATIONS: Due to the difficulty in internally using blue flag iris in a safe manner, I recommend it only for external use. Oil infusions and decoctions of the dried root are recommended. Cooled decoctions of the root can be preserved with witch hazel applied as an astringent, while the oil can be used to moisturize.

HERBAL SUBSTITUTES: Burdock (*Arctium lappa*): acne

SAFETY AND PRECAUTIONS

Avoid fresh root. Do not use internally unless under the supervision of an herbal practitioner. External use only.

LOOK-ALIKES: Sweet calamus (*Acorus calamus*), other Iris family members (*Iris* sp.) TOXIC

IDENTIFY & GROW

TYPE OF PLANT: Perennial (rhizome)

HABITAT: Blue flag irises prefer moist soils in moderate to full sun and are often seen grown along ditches and near waterways

HEIGHT: 2–3' (0.6–1 m)

LEAF: Long, thin strap-like foliage arising directly from the ground

FLOWER: Terminal deep blue-purple lipped flower with yellow coloring at the base of the sepal atop a long stem; appearing late spring through early summer

ROOT: Dense upright corm surrounded by many fibrous rootlets

GROWING INFORMATION: Plant rhizomes in areas that are uniformly cool and moist throughout the growing season, yet that receive full sun. Best planted along rocky ditches and swales and along waterway banks.

FORAGE OR GROW? Irises make for a stunning addition to the landscape. As such, blue flag iris is an herb to grow.

BEST HARVEST PRACTICES
ROOT HARVEST WINDOW: Early fall

Iris roots are best dug in early fall, then washed and sliced thinly to dry. It is advisable to wear gloves or limit your exposure to the juices of fresh-cut root.

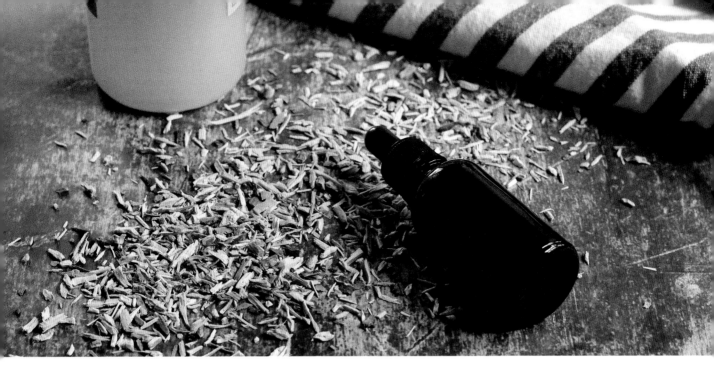

BLUE FLAG FACIAL OIL FOR ACNE-PRONE SKIN

A veteran of the skincare industry, I have long been singing the praises of facial oils.
Even for those with acne-prone skin.

(Audible gasp)

Yes, even acne-prone skin can benefit from a lightweight facial oil. Here blue flag iris is infused in light-weight jojoba oil which closely matches the lipid profile of human sebum, making it a nongreasy, light moisturizer. Once fully absorbed, jojoba oil leaves no trace of greasy residue and leaves skin feeling plump and soft. The healing and clearing benefits of blue flag iris are highlighted in this formula, promising smoother and clearer skin with patience and regular use. The optional addition of helichrysum essential oil adds further healing and scar prevention.

YIELD: 4 ounces (120 ml)

INGREDIENTS

4 oz (120 ml) jojoba oil

¼ cup (30 g) dried blue flag iris root

24 drops helichrysum essential oil (optional)

INSTRUCTIONS

Using either the regular or heated oil infusion method (page 12), infuse the jojoba oil with blue flag iris root. When the infusion is complete, strain the oil through double layers of flour sack cloth into a small bowl or liquid measuring cup. Add the helichrysum essential oil, if desired. Pour into two 2-ounce (60-ml) amber glass dropper bottles.

To use the facial oil, add 10 to 15 drops of the oil into the palms of your hands. Warm by rubbing your hands gently together and pat onto a clean, towel-dry face. Oil should be fully absorbed in a matter of minutes, without leaving a greasy shine. Use within 1 year.

COTTONWOOD

OTHER COMMON NAMES: western balsam-popular, black cottonwood, California poplar

LATIN NAME: *Populus trichocarpa* or *P. balsamifera*

HERBAL ENERGETICS: cool/dry

THERAPEUTIC ACTIONS: analgesic, anti-inflammatory, antimicrobial, astringent, diaphoretic, expectorant, vulnerary

PARTS USED: spring buds, leaves, inner bark

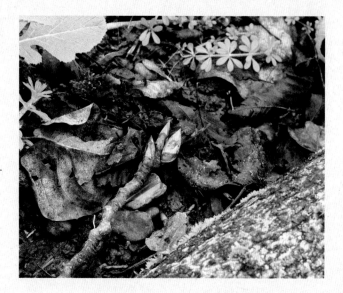

HERBAL MONOGRAPH

The aroma of cottonwood is the defining scent of many low-lying areas and waterways. Its sweet perfume is reminiscent of honey. Not coincidentally, industrious early season bees collect the resinous exudate from late winter buds for propolis production. Cottonwood buds were some of my earliest foraging conquests. Often appearing toward the end of winter, foraging buds is the perfect herbal escapism from housebound life during long, damp and dark winters. I find the process of locating windfallen branches and picking their swollen buds incredibly meditative, if a bit messy. Just me and the early birds, and if I am early enough, I don't even have to wade through seas of blackberries and nettle to gather my haul.

Cottonwood is ancient medicine. We even see reference to it or to a related species as balm of Gilead—a healing salve worthy of mention in a book of miracles. In a book in which seas get parted and water turns into wine, balm of Gilead had to be some pretty powerful stuff. This is not to say that cottonwood is a miracle herb, but it is a profoundly effective and highly medicinal herb with an abundance of therapeutic applications. As balm of Gilead, cottonwood is an extraordinary wound-healing herb, helping skin to mend and preventing infections associated with scrapes and cuts, while also relieving pain associated with deep tissue bruising and minor burns. Perhaps its chief therapeutic action is really the relief of residual inflammation at the site of trauma or injury by decreasing swelling and stagnation.

Due to the aspirin-like compounds, I tend to think of cottonwood as an herb for pain relief and fever management. Prepared as a salve with warming herbs, cottonwood promotes pain relief in aching joints and stodgy, tight muscles by increasing blood flow to the area of application. I find this to induce a wonderful warming sensation followed by a sense of coolness coupled with lasting relief. While it isn't always advisable for a holistic standpoint (you may want to let a low-grade fever run its course), a tincture of cottonwood can be very helpful in arresting a persistent high fever. As a diaphoretic, cottonwood encourages perspiration, which helps a fever to break by essentially expediting the running of its course. Do note that cottonwood is contraindicated for virally induced fevers such a chicken pox or the flu; it is more appropriate when used if fever is present with a bacterial infection such as strep throat.

Perhaps cottonwood's most understated medicinal virtue is that of expectorant. It is particularly useful when the throat is hot with glandular swelling and poor expectoration for fear of the pain coughing causes. It is also a specific herb for laryngitis and most throat complaints resulting in an alteration of the voice, such as loss of voice and hoarseness. By relieving pain and swelling, cottonwood helps propel the proverbial "junk" more efficiently out of the upper respiratory system.

TIP: When harvesting cottonwood buds, it is advisable to wear gloves in order to prevent sticky finger.

BEST PREPARATIONS: Teas can be produced with inner bark or leaves. Early spring buds can be infused into oil for massage or for salve making. Tinctures of cottonwood bud require a higher percentage of alcohol to fully extract the resinous constituents. I recommend the use of 195 proof spirits, sometimes referred to as Everclear.

HERBAL SUBSTITUTES: Willow (*Salix* sp.)

SAFETY AND PRECAUTIONS
It is best to avoid cottonwood remedies if taking blood-thinning medications or herbs, pregnant or nursing. As cottonwood contains methyl salicylate (the same active constituent in aspirin), do not use if you have an aspirin allergy or with conditions in which aspirin use is contraindicated, such as chicken pox and influenza (especially flu "B").

LOOK-ALIKES: *Populus* sp.

IDENTIFY & GROW

🌸 **TYPE OF PLANT:** Deciduous tree

🌸 **HABITAT:** Usually found near waterways such as streams, ponds and rivers—anywhere water is present. Cottonwood is quite often found in mixed forest with alder, willow species and maple nearby.

🌸 **HEIGHT:** 60–100' (18–30 m)

🌸 **LEAF:** Brownish red, resinous buds precede catkins in late winter. Mature leaves are simple and heart-shaped.

🌸 **STEM/LIMB:** Limbs and outer twigs are brittle and knobby.

🌸 **TRUNK:** Bark on young trees is smooth with a yellow-green cast, while older bark is brown-gray, craggy and almost cork-like. Root system is often quite shallow.

🌸 **FLOWER:** Pendulous catkins appear in early spring

🌸 **SEED:** Seeds are carried in a cottony fuzz that blows from the trees in mid-spring

🌸 **FORAGE OR GROW?** I would not advise planting cottonwoods in close proximity to one's home as they tend to suffer from strong winds and storms. This is an herb to forage.

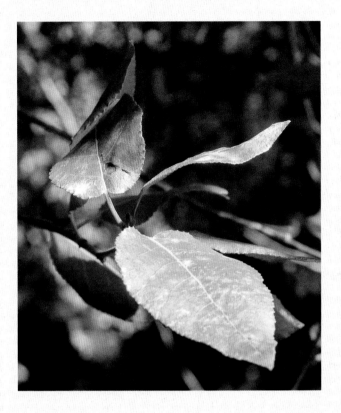

BEST HARVEST PRACTICES
BUD HARVEST WINDOW: Late winter through early spring

Forage buds and bark from windfall near local waterway after storms. Do not overharvest from live limbs, especially in younger trees as this might kill it. You may want to wear nitrile gloves when harvesting buds as they exude a sticky resin that is difficult to wash off. If buds are heavily soiled, rinse lightly; dry all buds before storage as excessive moisture content can cause the buds to mold. I find the buds store best when dried until the resin is solid and brittle—not sticky. Inner bark can be peeled and stripped from young limbs and dried.

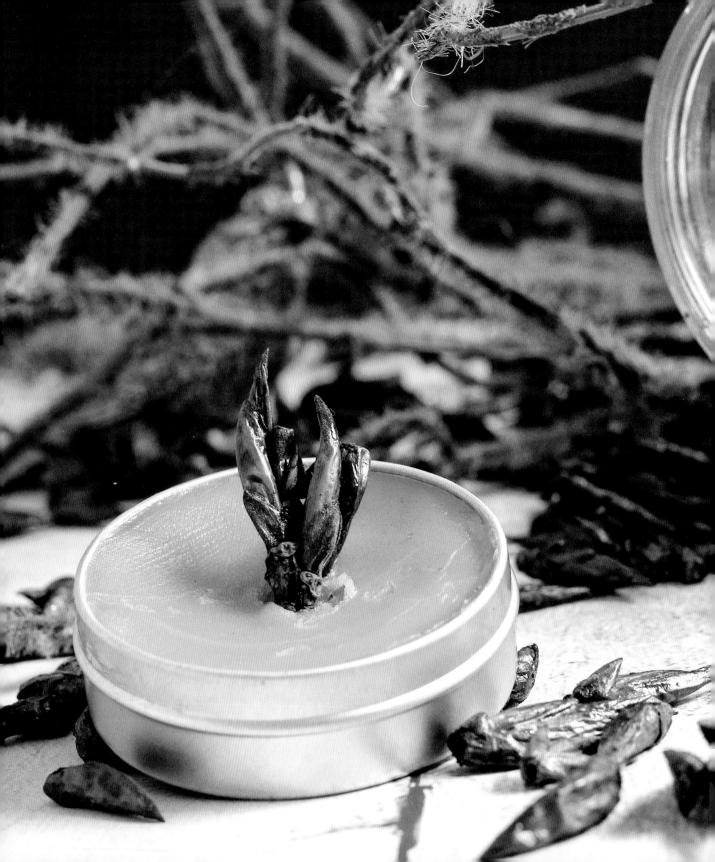

COTTONWOOD SALVE FOR ACHY, ANGRY JOINTS

Cottonwood is known for its wound healing benefits courtesy of its balm of Gilead fame, but it is an exceptional herb for sore, arthritic joints and tender muscles. Combined with the intense warming action of cayenne, this salve speeds healing blood flow to painful areas, delivering speedy relief from pain. Within 20 minutes of application of this salve, I always experience profound and quantifiable pain relief.

YIELD: approximately 8 ounces (240 ml)

INGREDIENTS

½ cup (50 g) dried cottonwood buds

1 tbsp (7 g) cayenne pepper flakes

1 cup (235 ml) base oil blend of your choice (I like coconut oil and olive oil here)

2–4 tbsp (20–40 g) beeswax pastilles

INSTRUCTIONS

Using the heated oil infusion method (page 12), infuse the cottonwood buds and cayenne into the base oils. After the oil is adequately infused, strain through muslin or cheese cloth. Return the oil to a double boiler, add the beeswax and warm until completely melted. Remove the oil-beeswax mixture from the heat.

Pour into individual 2-ounce (60-ml) containers, approximately 4, or other similarly sized jars. Allow to cool completely before putting a lid on the container. Apply to sore and stiff areas as needed. Use within 1 year.

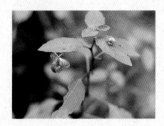

JEWELWEED

OTHER COMMON NAMES: touch-me-not, silverleaf

LATIN NAME: *Impatiens capensis*

HERBAL ENERGETICS: cool/moist

THERAPEUTIC ACTIONS: antihistamine, anti-inflammatory

PARTS USED: aboveground parts

HERBAL MONOGRAPH

Such a fitting name: jewelweed. It is a glowing punctuation mark in the wooded shade. A bright orange beacon, radiating a sunny glow underneath the canopy. Jewelweed is often found growing among the botanical for which it is the most traditional remedy: poison ivy.

Jewelweed is an age-old remedy for the painful, irritating rashes associated with exposure to poison oak, poison ivy and poison sumac (not to be confused with the similarly named sumacs of the *Rhus* genus). Scientific consensus is mixed about jewelweed's efficacy against urushiol—the rash-causing constituent of the aforementioned offenders. It is an anecdotal favorite that has been used for urushiol-induced contact dermatitis for years. I would argue that the efficacy of jewelweed is all about the timing of application. Jewelweed seems to be most effective when applied after exposure, but before the characteristic rash appears. Obviously, this particular type of efficacy is hard to quantify. After the rash appears, most herbalists observe that jewelweed helps to mitigate the severity of the symptoms and control the spread of the rash. Jewelweed seems to work best when exposed skin is thoroughly washed and dried, then has the fresh juice of jewelweed applied to the exposed area. When addressing these urushiol-induced rashes, avoid any oil-based jewelweed preparations as the oil may cause the rash to spread.

You might find this herbal monograph rather short and sweet compared to other botanicals in this book. There is some argument of the toxicity of jewelweed when used internally. Large doses are known to cause vomiting. That being said, jewelweed's admirable urushiol-fighting characteristics bear inclusion as one of my favorite forage-able plants.

BEST PREPARATIONS: Jewelweed is best prepared "juiced" with enough water to make it a liquid, otherwise known as a succus. Due to the rapid degradation of such a fresh preparation, succuses can be frozen in ice cube trays for future use.

HERBAL SUBSTITUTES: Calendula (*Calendula officinalis*)

SAFETY AND PRECAUTIONS

There are no known safety risks when using jewelweed externally. Internal use is not advised. Please seek out medical care if a rash becomes severe.

LOOK-ALIKES: Clearweed (*Pilea pumila*)

IDENTIFY & GROW

TYPE OF PLANT: Annual

HABITAT: Jewelweed prefers the deep shade of a forested area with deep, moist soils. It is often observed near poison ivy as it prefers the same habitat.

HEIGHT: 3–5' (1–1.5 m)

LEAF: Green ovoid leaves with moderately toothed margins. Lower leaves are arranged in opposite pairs, while upper leaves move to an alternate spacing. Leaves have a silvery underside.

STEM: Thin, hairless, waterfilled with swollen nodes

FLOWER: Somewhat tubular yellow to orange flowers with red spots with a modified sepal creating a "pouch" appearing June through early September

SEED: Small seed capsule; bursts when touched, issuing an audible popping sound

GROWING INFORMATION: Jewelweed seeds should be cold stratified and sown directly into moist, humus-rich soil in a shady area after all danger of frost has passed. Will reseed readily under proper conditions.

FORAGE OR GROW? Jewelweed offers a delicate and beautiful pop of color in the back of a shady herbaceous border, making this botanical a lovely addition to the garden. It is also easily identified in its natural habitat. This botanical is suited to either growing or foraging.

BEST HARVEST PRACTICES
ABOVEGROUND PARTS HARVEST WINDOW: Summer

Harvest aboveground parts of the plants and prepare fresh.

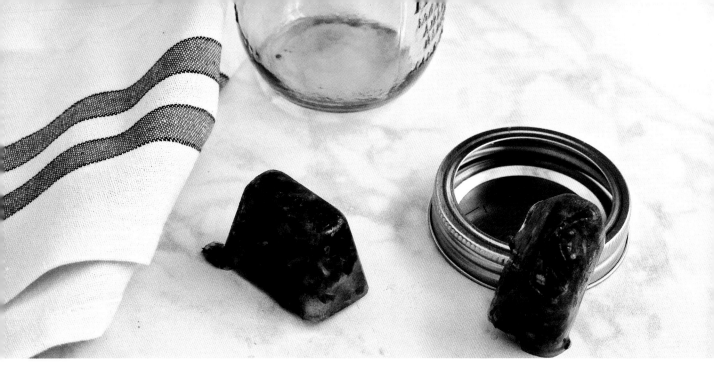

JEWELWEED SUCCUS FOR POISON IVY/OAK/SUMAC RASHES

This is a classic case where the simplest remedy is the best recipe. The first line of defense in any poison ivy/oak/sumac rash is to make sure that the exposed area is washed thoroughly with soap and water and rinsed well. All exposed clothing should be washed as well. This succus is basically just jewelweed that has been juiced with a small amount of water or aloe vera (for some extra soothing benefit) and applied to the skin. I haven't provided measurements, as this is such a recipe that you really must "eyeball"—adding just the tiniest bit of liquid to the blender until you have a good loose slurry of pureed herbs and liquid. Freeze the succus in ice cube trays for a ready supply of this handy botanical when needed.

YIELD: varies

INGREDIENTS

Jewelweed

Water or aloe vera juice

INSTRUCTIONS

In a small blender, blend the jewelweed until it is well chopped. Start adding a small amount of water or aloe vera, pulsing between each addition until you have a loose slurry of herb and liquid. Pour into ice cube molds and freeze. After freezing in trays, pop out and store in zip-closure bags in the freezer. Use within 1 year.

To use, thaw out a cube and apply to exposed or affected skin. Allow the succus to dry on the skin, and wipe off the herbs when dried.

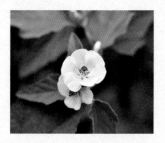

MARSHMALLOW

OTHER COMMON NAMES: althea, cheeses, sweet weed

LATIN NAME: *Althea officinalis*

HERBAL ENERGETICS: cool/moist

THERAPEUTIC ACTIONS: antibacterial, anti-inflammatory, antitussive, demulcent, diuretic (mild), hypoglycemic, immunostimulant, nutritive, vulnerary

PARTS USED: roots, leaves and flowers to a lesser degree but still quite mucilage rich

---

HERBAL MONOGRAPH

Marshmallow is the cooling, soothing oasis for all matters of hot and dry conditions. Inside and out, marshmallow calms the flames of inflammation and irritation with swiftness and efficacy.

Where there is heat, marshmallow stands and delivers. It is a choice herb for hot, dry respiratory conditions, soothing inflammation and coating fragile, practically friable mucus membranes. It also delivers infection-fighting properties, best used as a supportive adjunct when infection is a concern. As such, marshmallow is ideally suited for hot, dry complaints of the mouth, throat, stomach and digestive tract. It is an indispensable herb for sore throats and swollen glands associated with laryngitis, pharyngitis and generalized, chronic bronchitis.

More than an herb for sore throats, marshmallow offers great soothing and healing benefits for the digestive system. Much as observed with hot conditions of the respiratory systems, marshmallow also brings relief to complaints of heartburn, GERD, ulcers, indigestion and gastroenteritis. This herb may also aid in the management of diverticulitis and help expedite the healing of rectal fissures. It is particularly well suited to restoring the mucosal barrier during bouts of diarrhea, while also promoting a healthy balanced gut.

Marshmallow's benefits are not limited to internal complaints. It is a particularly amazing herb to address hot, red, inflamed skin conditions. Cool compresses of marshmallow root can bring practically immediate relief to the surface redness and irritation associated with rosacea. It is excellent for chapped, fragile skin experienced from rashes, wind and sunburn. It is ideal for even the most sensitive of skin.

BEST PREPARATIONS: For internal uses, marshmallow is best prepared as a cold infusion. Warm teas and infusions should be prepared with the bare minimum of heat to preserve as much of the soothing mucilage as possible. Cold-infused oils offer soothing anti-inflammatory action.

HERBAL SUBSTITUTES: Many members of the Malavaceae family can be used interchangeably including hibiscus (*Hibiscus militaris*), hollyhock (*Althea rosea*), common mallow (*Malva neglecta*) and rose of Sharon (*Hibiscus syriacus*).

SAFETY AND PRECAUTIONS

Marshmallow can interfere with the absorption of some medications and should be avoided for at least 30 minutes prior to administration.

LOOK-ALIKES: Members of the Malvaceae family (most can be used somewhat interchangeably), cotton (*Gossypium hirsutum*) TOXIC

IDENTIFY & GROW

TYPE OF PLANT: Perennial

HABITAT: Marshmallow likes sunny locations (not the strong sun of late afternoon), with moist and rich soils. It is often found in sunny marshland, wet meadows, and can even be seen in brackish ditches near the seaside.

HEIGHT: 3–4' (1–1.2 m)

LEAF: Soft velvety, gray-green leaves with irregular serrated margins are palmate and slightly rounded

STEM: Tall central stem with leaf nodes arranged alternately

FLOWER: White to pink, five-petaled flowers often with a darker center with prominent pistil

ROOT: Long, thick, tapered and fibrous

GROWING INFORMATION: To ensure good germination, marshmallow seeds need to be cold stratified. After stratification, plant seeds in a well-mulched, evenly moist soil in a sunny, but relatively protected location.

FORAGE OR GROW? Wild, wetland areas are often fragile ecosystems that suffer from heavy traffic and disruption. Marshmallow is an herb to grow.

BEST HARVEST PRACTICES

LEAF AND FLOWER HARVEST WINDOW: Summer

ROOT HARVEST WINDOW: Fall

Marshmallow leaves and flowers can be harvested prior to blooming. Roots can be dug, cleaned and sliced for drying in early fall.

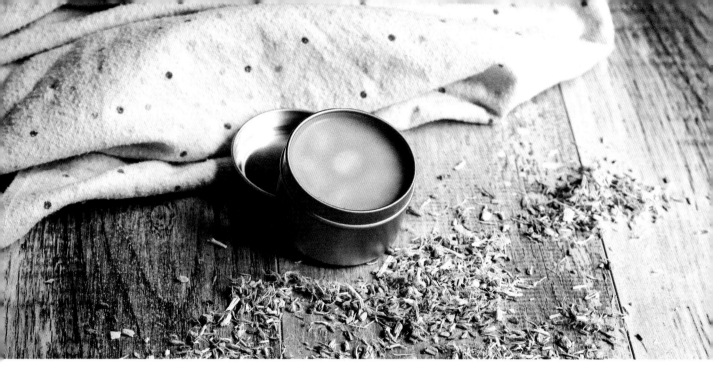

MARSHMALLOW BUM BALM FOR BOUNCING BABIES

Sweet little baby bums can become chapped and irritated so easily. Their sensitive skin deserves the gentlest of herbs. The soothing, cooling benefits of marshmallow are infused into a rich blend of oils to soften and heal tender bottoms.

Not limited to just babies, this balm is most excellent for other chafed and chapped skin in older individuals, such as experienced with "inner thigh rub" and irritation from athletic gear.

YIELD: approximately 8 ounces (240 ml)

INGREDIENTS

½ cup (15 g) dried marshmallow root

1 cup (235 ml) base oil blend of your choice (I like coconut oil and olive oil here)

2–4 tbsp (20–40 g) beeswax pastilles

INSTRUCTIONS

Using the regular or heated oil infusion method (page 12), infuse the marshmallow into the base oils. After the oil is adequately infused, strain through muslin or cheese cloth. Return the oil to a double boiler, add the beeswax and warm until completely melted. Remove the oil-beeswax mixture from the heat. Pour into individual 2-ounce (60-ml) containers, approximately 4, or other similarly sized jars. Allow to cool completely before putting a lid on the container.

Apply liberally to baby bum after each diaper change. This oil-based balm may stain cloth diapers and clothing. Use within 1 year.

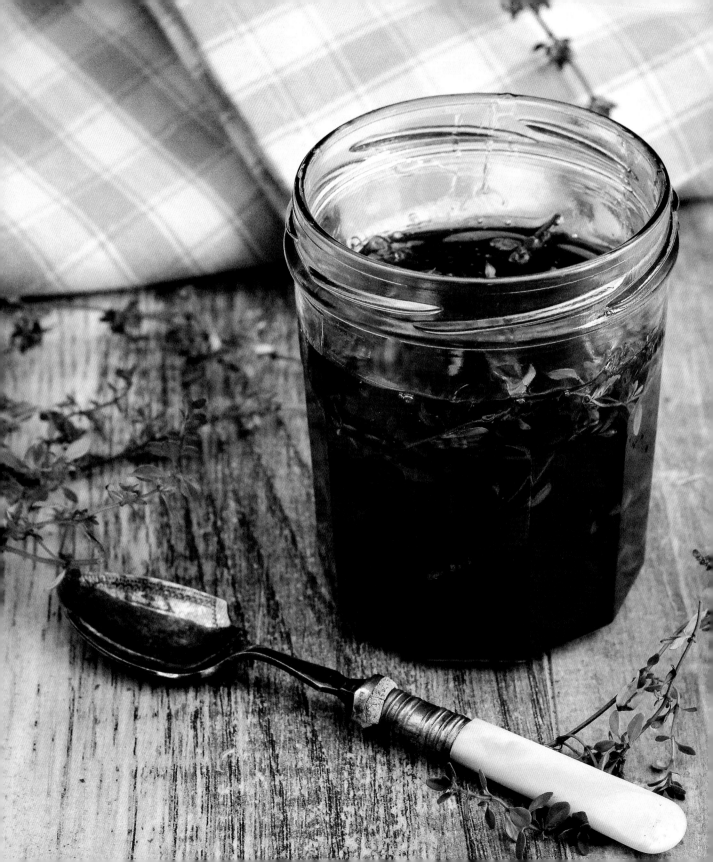

EASY TO GROW KITCHEN HERBS FOR NATURAL WELLNESS

MEDICINE IS EVERYWHERE. And the most important medicine, other than light and water, is food. In the garden we find nourishment in the form of fruits, vegetables and herbs. These common, almost everyday, botanicals are so often overlooked in favor of more elusive herbs, but they are some of the best medicines.

Just try to walk by tall spikes of rosemary without brushing your fingers through its camphor-y leaves, encouraging deep, lung-filling breaths. Indulge in the crisp, clean scent of lavender warmed by the sun to wash your worries away. Laugh and play with the sticky silks on every ear of corn, a soothing demulcent to calm inflammation. Make the most of your garden.

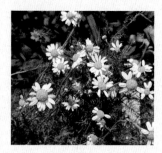

CHAMOMILE

OTHER COMMON NAMES: earth apple, maythen

LATIN NAME: *Matricaria recutita* (German chamomile), *Chamaemelum nobile* (Roman chamomile)

HERBAL ENERGETICS: cool/dry

THERAPEUTIC ACTIONS: antihistamine, anti-inflammatory, antispasmodic, carminative, diaphoretic, hypotensive, nervine, sedative, vulnerary

PARTS USED: flowering tops

HERBAL MONOGRAPH

Chamomile was the first herbal medicine that I knowingly used. Cursed with insomnia and restlessness from an early age, I probably learned of chamomile's sedative action from the front of a box of tea. Not exactly a reputable resource, but effective nonetheless. While the quality of those prebagged tea blends was certainly questionable in those days, chamomile's effect on my body wasn't. Calming and soothing, it not only eased me into sleep sooner, it helped me maintain a restful sleep that allowed me to awake refreshed. Quite a bit older and a little bit wiser now, I understand chamomile. It is the most grandmotherly of herbs—wholesome, soft, encouraging, capable of easing all your troubles.

As humans, our reductionist tendencies are to pigeonhole herbs by the disease that they are used to address. Chamomile is no exception: it seems to be associated with insomnia without fail. But insomnia isn't experienced in the same way by all sufferers. Some folks feel it too "in their head," with a busy brain too overworked to sleep. Chamomile may dial down the monkey brain for these individuals, but they will often require a more powerful sedative nervine, not to mention relaxation and coping techniques, to get the drop on insomnia. Others possess a body that holds sleep hostage. This is where I feel that chamomile really shines.

Beyond its mild sedative qualities, chamomile possesses a number of other therapeutic actions that promote relaxation. Chamomile is a highly effective antispasmodic, soothing aching muscles and releasing tense and tight smooth muscle tissue. Chamomile is like a slow release valve on the tension our bodies carry. It acts on the cardiovascular system, with both clinical and anecdotal evidence indicating that it can help to lower elevated blood pressure. Chamomile also serves as a carminative, dispelling the pressure of gas and bloating that often make relaxation impossible. It also cools the extremities, which promotes a more restful state. With these actions and its gentle sedative virtues, chamomile can usher the body into a restful slumber.

BEST PREPARATIONS: German chamomile makes for an excellent tea or infusion and can be tinctured fresh. Roman chamomile is preferable for oil infusions and aromatherapy due to a higher volatile oil content.

Chamomile is edible and has a flavor and aroma similar to green apple. It's a tasty addition to baked goods and liqueurs.

HERBAL SUBSTITUTES: Lavender (*Lavandula angustifolia*): nervine | hawthorn (*Crataegus* sp.): cardiovascular

SAFETY AND PRECAUTIONS

Do not use if you are allergic to members of the Asteraceae (daisy/ragweed) family. If you are pregnant, nursing or taking prescription medication, please consult your physician before taking this or any other herb.

LOOK-ALIKES: Pineapple weed (*Matricaria discoidea*)

IDENTIFY & GROW

TYPE OF PLANT: Perennial or free seeding annual

HABITAT: This low-growing botanical prefers full sun to light shade and well-drained soils.

HEIGHT: 1–2' (0.3–0.6 m)

LEAF: German chamomile has a fern-like leaf, while the Roman variety is a finely dissected, parsley-like leaf. Both emit a green apple odor.

FLOWER: Small white, daisy-like ray flower; appears late spring through the first frost

GROWING INFORMATION: Chamomile can be sown directly into soils after the danger of frost has passed. Soils should be fertile and well-drained. Keep evenly moist throughout establishment and water well during drought.

FORAGE OR GROW? Chamomile will often naturalize to areas given the right conditions, however this herb is one to grow.

BEST HARVEST PRACTICES
FLOWER HARVEST WINDOW: Summer

Harvest newly opened flowers throughout the blooming season and lay in a single layer to dry. Harvest frequently to promote new blooms.

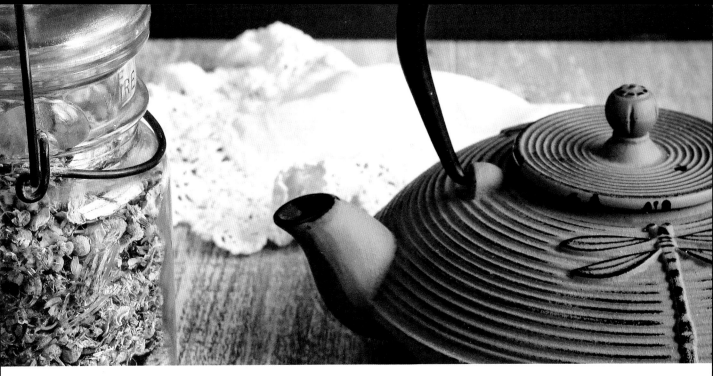

SLEEPY CHAMOMILE TEA BLEND FOR THE DREAMIEST SLUMBER

Most of us have experienced chamomile tea in our lifetime. It is a safe and gentle sleep aid that even little kids enjoy with its slightly apple-like flavor. I find that there is HUGE difference in quality among prebagged tea blends and prefer to mix my own. Chamomile should not smell musty or like wet cardboard; this is a sign that the chamomile is old or has not been dried properly. Always make sure that your chamomile has a pleasant odor of apple and dry hay.

I combine chamomile with a little bit of rose petals and lemon balm in this blend to promote a restful, pleasant slumber. The addition of lovely lavender is recommended, although some folks may find its flavor too soapy for their preferences. Just thinking about this tea makes the tension in my shoulders ease and my thoughts turn to the allure of my pillow. Pleasant dreams.

YIELD: a generous 3 cups (47 g) of dry blend

INGREDIENTS

1 cup (25 g) dried German chamomile flowers

½ cup (6 g) dried rose petals

½ cup (12 g) dried lemon balm

2 tbsp (4 g) dried lavender (optional)

INSTRUCTIONS

Mix the dried herbs well, and store in a jar with a tight-fitting lid in a cool, dark place. Use within 1 year.

To prepare the tea: Pour 8 to 10 ounces (240 to 300 ml) of water just off the boil over approximately 1 tablespoon (1 g) of this blend. Steep for 5 to 7 minutes, strain and serve. This tea is safe for adults and children.

LAVENDER

OTHER COMMON NAMES: English lavender, elf leaf, spikenard

LATIN NAME: *Lavandula angustifolia*

HERBAL ENERGETICS: cool/dry

THERAPEUTIC ACTIONS: antidepressant, anti-inflammatory, antimicrobial, antiseptic, antispasmodic, anxiolytic, astringent, carminative, cholagogue, hepatic, hypnotic, insect repellant, nervine, sedative, vulnerary

PARTS USED: flowering tops

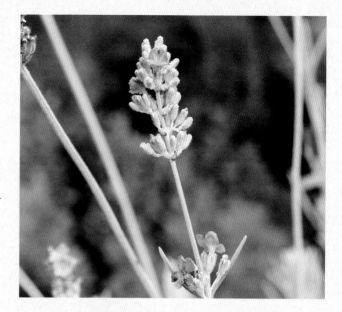

HERBAL MONOGRAPH

Ask me if I have a favorite child, and I will say, "Yes, but it changes with the hour." Ask me if I have a favorite herb, and I will probably blush and say "lavender" kind of sheepishly. My affinity for this botanical is profound.

There are other herbs. There are other flowers. And then there is lavender. Few other botanicals evoke such as sense of calm, beauty and peace. Whether dotted in a showy perennial border or placed into agricultural rows, lavender in full bloom is an experience to behold. Visually lovely, abuzz with pollinators and brimming with its clean, euphoric aroma, lavender is the fresh-faced beauty of the plant world. It is beloved by all—I don't trust those who can't abide a bit of lavender.

Lavender was one of the first herbs that I was determined to grow. In my early teen years, those first seeds planted in flimsy seed starting trays failed miserably, overwatered and squashed by the cat. A few gardens later, I finally started producing those showy plants that I so admired. I can never pass a lavender spike without running my fingers through the foliage and buds. To me, lavender is practically the perfect plant.

Lavender is well known, especially in the aromatherapy field, for its ability to uplift one's spirits. This herb has a long and storied history of being used to prevent quarrelsome behavior, deter evil from the household and even keep monks and nuns chaste and holy. Much in the way that lavender is associated with cleanliness of our physical places and things, I would suggest that lavender contributes to cleanliness of the mind. It seems to sweep out the mental clutter that contributes to insomnia, lack of concentration, tension headaches and argumentative behavior. Lavender keeps everybody cool, calm and collected.

In another nod to the "cleanliness" of lavender, it is a well-regarded herb for skin and wound care. With antimicrobial and antiseptic action, lavender is well suited to wound sprays and salves, helping to guard against infection and necrotic tissue. Lavender is especially well suited to addressing the discomforts associated with burns. Its cooling anti-inflammatory actions provides soothing relief to sunburns and contact burns. Lavender is also used as an herbal bug repellant deterring lice and mosquitoes. It is a popular addition to skincare routines helping to normalize oil production, decrease redness and calm itchy scalps.

Just as lavender relaxes the mind and calms the skin, this herb soothes tense and spasmodic muscles. Lavender loosens the tight knots produced from overwork and tension, while also soothing menstrual, stomach and bowel cramping. This herb provides lasting relaxation, and it is perfect for clearing the path to a good night's rest.

BEST PREPARATIONS: Both the leaves and flowers of lavender are high in aromatic oils and relaxing constituents. Although flowers are most likely to be seen in commercial preparations, I do not object to the use of leaves gathered during the lavender harvest. Waste not, want not!

Lavender lends itself well to teas and infusions, often combining well with mints or chamomile to offset its somewhat soapy flavor. Tinctures of lavender are especially helpful for internal cramping. Base oils infused with dried lavender for salve making and for massage are most delightful. Lavender essential oil is gentle enough that it can be applied neat (without dilution), although a patch test is suggested. Lavender hydrosol can be misted onto sheets to promote restful sleep or spritzed onto laundry for a sense of cleanliness.

Lavender makes a lovely edible flower when treated with a slight hand. The herb can be infused into sugar or honey, added to baked goods and added to the classic French herbes de Provence. I even infuse a few springs of lavender into my annual blueberry jam.

HERBAL SUBSTITUTES: Chamomile (*Matricaria recutita*): sedative | calendula (*Calendula officinalis*): vulnerary

SAFETY AND PRECAUTIONS
Lavender is largely considered safe in normal amounts. If you are pregnant, nursing or taking prescription medication, please consult your physician before taking this or any other herb.

LOOK-ALIKES: Other *Lavandula* species

IDENTIFY & GROW
TYPE OF PLANT: Perennial

HABITAT: Lavender likes bright, sunny locations with sandy, well-drained soils. It is tolerant of somewhat dry conditions.

HEIGHT: 2–3' (0.6–1 m)

LEAF: Silvery, gray-green, narrow lance-shaped leaves about 1" (2.5 cm) in length arranged in whorls

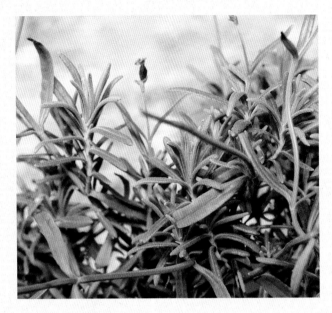

STEM: The stem arises from whorled leaves and becomes bare before being topped with a flower spike.

FLOWER: Long-lasting spikes of small purple flowers; appear early summer and mature throughout the growing season

GROWING INFORMATION: Lavender seeds can be started indoors and transplanted outside after all danger of frost has passed. Plant seedlings or young plants in an area of full sun and light soils. Lavender plants need plenty of air circulation and are tolerant of drought-like conditions after establishment.

FORAGE OR GROW? Lavender doesn't often naturalize to landscapes, making this herb most appropriate for planting in the home garden.

BEST HARVEST PRACTICES
FLOWERING TOPS HARVEST WINDOW: Summer

Harvest flowering stems just as the flower buds begin to open and dry adequately. Leaves are also highly aromatic and can be used as well.

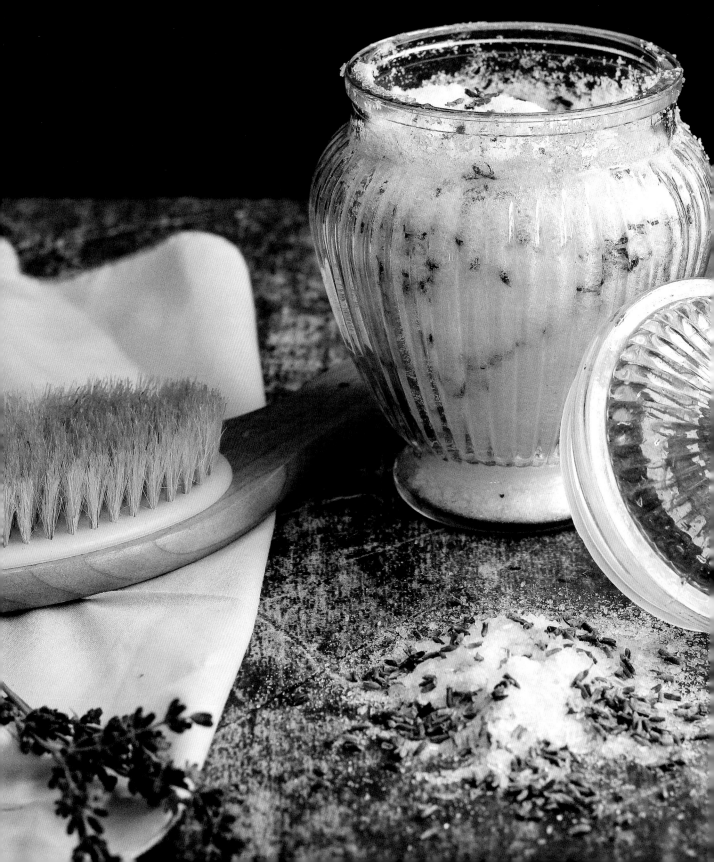

RESTORATIVE LAVENDER BATH SOAK FOR TIRED & TENSE BEINGS

There is hardly anything more relaxing than a lavender-scented tub full of warm, steamy water and soft lighting. After busy days, tight deadlines, persnickety customers, harsh lighting and nonstop stress, we all deserve a little relaxation.

This bath soak harnesses the great relaxing energies of lavender and Epsom salts and adds skin-softening moisture courtesy of sweet almond oil. A soak in this blend loosens those tight neck muscles and releases tension headaches while nourishing your skin and body.

YIELD: 4 cups (about 860 g)

INGREDIENTS

3½ cups (840 g) Epsom salts

½ cup (15 g) dried lavender buds

2 tbsp (30 ml) sweet almond oil

20 drops lavender essential oil (optional)

INSTRUCTIONS

In a medium-sized bowl, combine all the ingredients until well distributed. Transfer into decorative jars for storage until use. Use within 1 year.

To use, add 1 to 2 cups (215 to 430 g) of the mixture to your bathtub while the water is filling, swirling around to help the mixture dissolve. Soak for at least 10 to 20 minutes.

NOTE: Be very careful upon standing, as the tub may be slick from the sweet almond oil. Rinse the tub well after using.

CALENDULA

OTHER COMMON NAMES: pot marigold, bride of the sun
LATIN NAME: *Calendula officinalis*
HERBAL ENERGETICS: neutral/neutral
THERAPEUTIC ACTIONS: anti-inflammatory, antimicrobial, antispasmodic, astringent, demulcent, emmenagogue, hepatic, lymphatic, vulnerary
PARTS USED: flowers

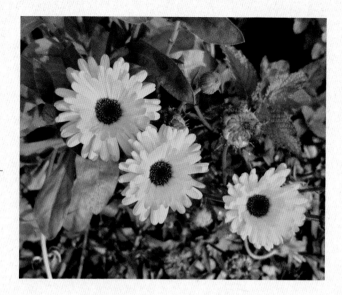

HERBAL MONOGRAPH

Calendula has a place in every home apothecary. It is, very simply put, an amazing herb. Many of us learned about calendula early on in our herbal studies. It is a gateway herb. Once you understand the many virtues of this sunny little flower, the wide world of healing botanicals is yours to benefit from. Calendula shines a radiant light on the world of herbs. What's not to love about the vibrant flowers in shades of yellow and orange that bloom all summer long, providing harvests of their sticky, resinous blooms? Calendula is a gift from Mother Nature in more ways than one.

For many of us, calendula became part of our herbal knowledge foundation as a "first aid" botanical. It is one of the best regarded herbs for all kinds of trauma and injury. As a chief vulnerary herb, calendula not only mends broken skin, it relieves inflammation and minimizes the formation of scar tissue. It is so effective in closing minor wounds that it should only be applied when no infection is present (or applied in conjunction with a stronger antimicrobial herb), as the skin may "seal" over the infection. It is ideally used for minor cuts, scratches, blisters and bruising with inflammation. Liberal use of calendula-based remedies will keep a wound soft and pliable.

Calendula is a go-to herb for a variety of skin complaints. It is the perfect herb for soothing chapped skin due to wind, sun or friction burns—providing calming relief to the redness and irritation. As such it is an excellent herb for bedsores and blisters, as well as nipple, inner thigh and groin area chafing. It also relieves itching, making it a comfort for fever-y rashes and contact dermatitis. Calendula relieves the pain, redness and scarring associated with deep, hormonally triggered sebaceous cysts. Some resources point to calendula for softening the appearance of freckles and reducing excessive facial hair.

Calendula is often undervalued as a lymphatic tonic. It is recommended when there are complaints of hardened and inflamed lymph nodes, particularly around the neck, underarm and groin. As such, it is suggested for underarm complaints, such as sensitivity and odor, pulling triple duty by softening skin, mitigating unattractive scents and very possibly slowing the growth of underarm hair.

Due to its dual properties of being both astringent and demulcent, calendula makes an extraordinary herb for complaints of the digestive system. It helps to tone lax tissue, arrest fluid loss and minor internal bleeding and provides a protective barrier for the gastric mucosal lining. Calendula is suggested when one is suffering from heartburn and acid reflux, as well as gastric, duodenal and peptic ulcers.

BEST PREPARATIONS: Such a versatile herb can be prepared in a variety of ways. Infused oils make for an excellent massage, lotion/cream and salve-making base. Cooled water-based infusion can be sprayed onto inflamed skin or applied as a compress. A poultice of calendula may be effective for blisters and warts. For internal use, teas, tinctures and infusions may provide lasting relief. Calendula tinctures (for internal use or witch hazel infusions for external use) are best made with fresh plant material.

Calendula petals are edible with a bland floral flavor. These can be added to salads and baked goods, and used as edible floral garnishes. Petals are sometimes used as an inexpensive alternative to saffron for coloring dishes. One should note the flavor, however, is not the same.

HERBAL SUBSTITUTES: Yarrow (*Achillea millefolium*): antimicrobial, astringent

SAFETY AND PRECAUTIONS
Do not use if you are allergic to members of the Asteraceae (daisy/ragweed) family. If you are pregnant, nursing or taking prescription medication, please consult a physician before using this or any other herb.

LOOK-ALIKES: False sunflower (*Heliopsis helianthoides*), gerber daisy (*Gerbera jamesonii*) TOXIC to some pets and livestock

IDENTIFY & GROW
  TYPE OF PLANT: Annual

  HABITAT: Calendula prefers sunny spots with well-drained soils.

  HEIGHT: 12–24" (30–60 cm)

  LEAF: Simple, green, alternate leaves

  STEM: Hairy

  FLOWER: Ray-like petals radiate around a central disk of the small tubular "flower" like many members of the daisy family. Yellow and orange flowers may be single or double.

  SEED: Interesting, arched "serpent-y" looking seeds

  GROWING INFORMATION: Start seeds indoors 6 to 8 weeks before the last expected frost for your area. Transplant outside when all danger of frost has passed.

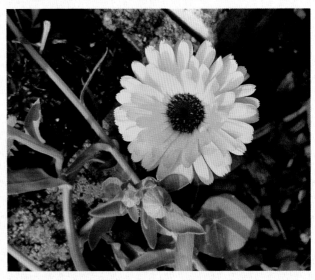

Water often and top dress with nutrient-rich compost throughout the growing season. Pick flowers or deadhead for repeat blooms, leaving the last of the season's flowers to go to seed to encourage next year's growth.

  FORAGE OR GROW? Calendula is not considered a "wild" herb, but it can quickly naturalize in an area and become quite feral. If such a patch exists near you, this is prime foraging material. However, calendula grows easily from seed or transplant and is easily cared for in the home garden. Additionally, calendula is a popular companion plant, encouraging beneficial insects and pollinators, while reducing pests and disease in the garden.

BEST HARVEST PRACTICES
FLOWER HARVEST WINDOW: Summer to early fall (often flowers continuously until frost)

Harvest calendula just as the buds start to open and dry thoroughly. Some herbalists prefer to remove petals from the calyx to ensure the calendula is properly dry, whereas others feel the resinous calyx should remain.

CALENDULA PIT PASTE FOR THE SWEETEST UNDERARMS

There is no question that commercial deodorant and antiperspirants often have some real eyebrow-raising ingredients. Many of us have made the switch to an all-natural DIY deodorant only to experience a fiery hell pit due to the inclusion of baking soda. It's all well and good until one day your pit starts itching and itching and ITCHING! Many will consider their hike into the ultimate in crunchy living territory failed in this holy grail of DIY personal care items.

But luckily, baking soda isn't altogether necessary, especially when you combine a few thoughtfully planned ingredients with calendula-infused oil. Calendula supports good lymphatic health and minimizes funky smelling bacteria, leaving you with soft, silky and sweet pits. This two-part recipe makes more calendula-infused oil than is necessary for the pit paste batch. Save this oil for salve making and for massage.

YIELD: approximately 8–10 ounces (240–300 ml)

CALENDULA-INFUSED OIL

2 cups (480 ml) base oil(s) of your choosing (I like a 50/50 combination of coconut oil and sweet almond oil here.)

1 cup (15 g) dried calendula flowers

PIT PASTE

½ cup (120 ml) calendula-infused oil

1 oz (30 g) cocoa, mango or shea butter

2 oz (20 g) beeswax pastilles

2 tbsp (30 g) arrowroot powder

2 tbsp (30 g) kaolin clay

20–40 drops essential oils of your choice, optional (some of my favorites are lavender, geranium, sweet orange, cedarwood and sage)

CALENDULA-INFUSED OIL

Prepare the calendula-infused oil using one of the methods described on page 12. Strain through two layers of flour sack cloth into a liquid measuring cup or jar. Reserve the oil in excess of what is needed for this recipe in a jar for massage or for salve making. Store in a cool, dark place and use within 1 year.

PIT PASTE

Combine the calendula-infused oil, cocoa butter and beeswax into the top bowl of a double boiler. Heat gently until melted and well combined. Remove from the heat; quickly add the arrowroot, kaolin clay and optional essential oils and stir continuously until the mixture is slightly thickened but still pourable. Pour into small 2-ounce (60-ml) tins or disposable deodorant tube blanks. Allow to fully cool before capping.

Pit paste can be applied with clean fingers if using tins, or normally if using deodorant tube blanks. Some people may find it necessary to reapply a couple times throughout the day, at least when transitioning to a homemade deodorant. Over time, the bacteria load of the underarm and your lymphatic health will improve, decreasing the necessity for reapplication. Use within 1 year.

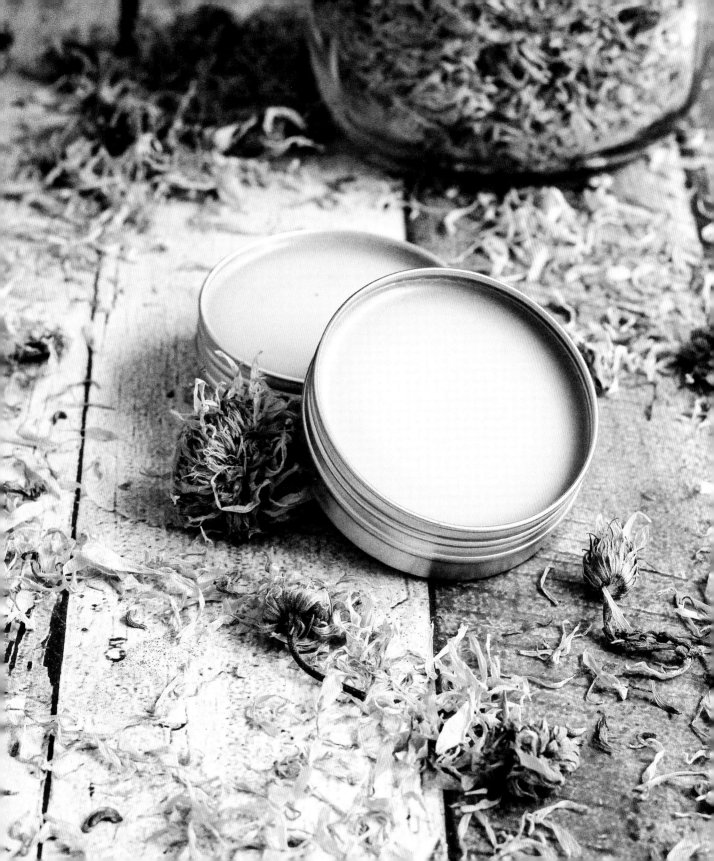

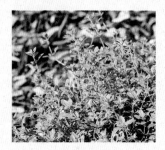

THYME

OTHER COMMON NAMES: farigoule, seprolet

LATIN NAME: *Thymus vulgaris*

HERBAL ENERGETICS: hot/dry

THERAPEUTIC ACTIONS: anthelmintic, anti-inflammatory, antimicrobial, antioxidant, antiseptic, antispasmodic, astringent, carminative, diaphoretic, diffusive, emmenagogue, expectorant, stimulant

PARTS USED: leaves, flowering tops

HERBAL MONOGRAPH

If there was one herb that I simply could not do without in my cooking, it would surely be thyme. While thyme might seem like the grandmother of kitchen herbs, it is really the unsung superhero of culinary-medicinal herbs. Simply put, thyme makes you feel better—just like grandma.

Thyme is a truly antiseptic herb. Most people think of "antiseptics" as translating to "antibacterial" or "germ-fighting." However, the medical definition of antiseptic expands on the antimicrobial aspects to include actions that prevent "sepsis, putrefaction and decay," according to Merriam-Webster. Thyme plays an important role in wound care. Thyme washes, compresses and salves can be used to address bed sores and other friction-related ulcerations, as well as cuts and abrasions. Thyme essential oil has also been shown in studies to be effective against methicillin-resistant *Staphylococcus aureus* bacterial infection, as well as the bacteria that cause topical acne.

Thyme is very well suited to cold, damp conditions of the upper respiratory system. As an aromatic and warming herb, it helps to thin thick mucus and bronchial secretions, allay spasmodic coughing fits and fight infection. As such, it is a useful herb for fighting complaints of whooping cough, asthma and bronchitis. Thyme also is extremely soothing for abdominal complaints, such as nausea due to sinus drainage, colic, bloating and gas.

BEST PREPARATIONS: Thyme is an herb that I use both fresh and dried. It makes a warming, woodsy tea or infusion. Clothes can be soaked in a cool thyme infusion to wash wounds and sores. Dried thyme–infused oils can be prepared into wound care salves. The herb can also be infused into distilled vinegar to wash surfaces and spray onto suspect fresh vegetables and fruits; rinse before eating.

Thyme is an excellent herb for culinary purposes. One of my favorite meals involves slathering a roasting chicken with seasoned thyme compound butter, and roasting it on a bed of new red potatoes. Perfection.

HERBAL SUBSTITUTES: Bee balm (*Monarda* sp.): diffusive

SAFETY AND PRECAUTIONS

Thyme is safe as used in food. Use extreme caution when using thyme essential oil as it can "burn" the mucosa and sensitive tissues. If you are pregnant, nursing or taking prescription medication, please contact your physician before using this or any other herb.

LOOK-ALIKES: Wild basil (*Clinopodium vulgare*)

IDENTIFY & GROW

TYPE OF PLANT: Perennial

HABITAT: Thyme likes full sun and will thrive in poor soils and dry conditions.

HEIGHT: 6–12" (15–30 cm)

LEAF: Tiny leaves are somewhat ovoid and arranged opposite. Leaves may be solid green or variegated.

STEM: New growth is green and pliable, maturing to a woody stem.

FLOWER: Small, two-lipped, lilac pink flowers top stems; late spring to early summer

GROWING INFORMATION: Thyme seeds are notoriously recalcitrant about germinating, so cuttings are a more ideal means of propagation. Plant in full sun. Thyme thrives on neglect and is tolerant of drought conditions.

FORAGE OR GROW? Although wild thyme may be found in parts of Europe, it is not easily found outside of the garden elsewhere. Being that thyme is a "brown thumbed" gardener's dream come true, this is an herb to grow.

BEST HARVEST PRACTICES
FLOWERING TOP HARVEST WINDOW: Early summer

For medicinal purposes, the volatile oil content will be highest just as thyme begins to flower and dry. Thyme can be used fresh or dry for culinary purposes.

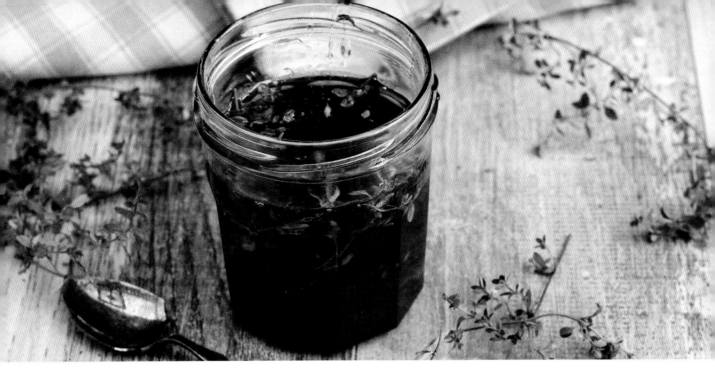

THYME-INFUSED HONEY FOR SORE THROATS & WET COUGHS

As I have stated before, simple remedies are the best remedies. Simple will always trump complicated recipes in my apothecary. It hardly gets simpler than thyme-infused honey. Thyme imparts the honey with its warming, stimulating action and its antimicrobial benefits, making this honey perfect for the wet coughs and sore throats of the cold season.

YIELD: 1 cup (240 ml)

ADULT/TEEN DOSE: 1 tbsp (15 ml), as needed

CHILD'S DOSE, AGES 6–12: 1 tsp, as needed

CHILD'S DOSE, AGES 2–5: ½ tsp, as needed

INGREDIENTS

10–15 sprigs fresh thyme

1 cup (240 ml) raw, unfiltered honey

INSTRUCTIONS

Coil freshly picked thyme sprigs around the bottom of a jar, packing as many sprigs in as seems reasonable. Pour honey over the thyme to cover. Infuse the honey with thyme for a minimum of 6 weeks, then strain through a fine-mesh sieve into a liquid measuring cup. Pour the infused honey into a jar for ease of use. This honey can be taken by the spoonful as needed or used to sweeten tea, when there are complaints of sore, irritated throats.

If kept from excessive moisture, this preparation will last indefinitely, although it may crystallize over time. Immerse the sealed jar into hot water to liquify. Discard if signs of mold or fermentation appear. This remedy can also be attractive to ants. Keep the jar well sealed. Use within 1 year.

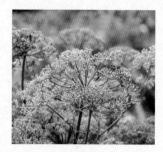

DILL

OTHER COMMON NAMES: dillweed, aneton

LATIN NAME: *Anethum graveolens*

HERBAL ENERGETICS: warm/dry

THERAPEUTIC ACTIONS: alterative, analgesic, antibacterial, antispasmodic, astringent, cardiovascular, carminative, diaphoretic, digestive, diuretic, emmenagogue, expectorant, galactagogue, nervine, sialagogue, stimulant

PARTS USED: seeds, leaf

HERBAL MONOGRAPH

You thought about pickles, didn't you? Perhaps it is with good reason. After all, dill is one of the most effective herbs for stimulating digestion. Dill is a strong sialagogue, meaning that it induces salivation. In doing so dill clears the palate and stimulates digestive function. As a warming herb, it promotes the concept of digestive fire, making it an ideal herb for those who have a predisposition to feeling tired and "dumpy" after a meal. As one of the most revered of carminative herbs, dill is a choice herb for dispelling gas, bloating and foul flatulence. And it acts quickly, providing almost immediate relief for gassy, eruptive indigestion. Additionally, it is a profoundly gentle colic reliever for suffering infants.

Dill is also an unexpected nervine herb. Some sources suggest that dill stimulates the parietal lobe of the brain, increasing navigative function, spatial awareness and sense of touch. It's ideal for those that feel "out of their head," "spaced out" and lacking attention to detail.

Where there are concerns of boggy sinuses, congestion and sneezing, dill offers a warm, stimulating jolt with its pungent aromatics. Ideally prepared as a steam, either in the form of a sauna or facial steam, it helps to release sinus pressure. Additionally, dill is a stimulating diaphoretic, promoting perspiration ideal for those with feverish chills and cold extremities.

BEST PREPARATIONS: Dill can be prepared as a tea, or the dried leaves or seeds can be chewed in a pinch. Fresh dill can also be tinctured. To maximize the digestive action of dill, the herb should be tasted, although a belly massage oil is also a suitable remedy for children. Dill is a wonderful culinary herb for pickles, eggs, fish and smoked and creamy foods.

HERBAL SUBSTITUTES: Fennel (*Foeniculum vulgare*): digestive

SAFETY AND PRECAUTIONS

If pregnant or trying to become pregnant, do not use more than amounts normally found in food, as members of this plant family (Apiaceae) are thought to have contraceptive and abortive action. If you are taking prescription medication, please consult your physician before taking this or any other herb.

LOOK-ALIKES: Fennel (*Foeniculum vulgare*)

IDENTIFY & GROW

TYPE OF PLANT: Annual

HABITAT: Dill likes sunny locations with well-drained soil and plenty of room to grow,

HEIGHT: 2–4' (0.6–1.2 m)

LEAF: Compound, alternate, finely cut, fern-y leaves with characteristic pungent aroma

FLOWER: Yellow umbels of tiny flowers appear mid- to late summer. Characteristic odor.

SEED: Small brown seeds mature late summer and do not split open when ripe.

GROWING INFORMATION: Dill does not respond well to transplant. Sow seeds into well-worked soil after all danger of frost has passed. Water frequently while establishing.

FORAGE OR GROW? Although feral stands of dill can be found along the Mediterranean and in a few other areas, it is an herb that most herbalist and chefs would suggest growing. Dill freely seeds if left to mature in the garden; expect lots of dill volunteers after your initial planting!

BEST HARVEST PRACTICES

LEAF/FROND HARVEST WINDOW: Summer

SEED HARVEST WINDOW: Late summer to fall

Leaves can be harvested throughout the growing season. If you want to gather seeds, do not trim foliage from the flowering stems. When seeds are brown and dry, cover each seed head with a paper bag, snip stalk and shake the flower head vigorously into the bag.

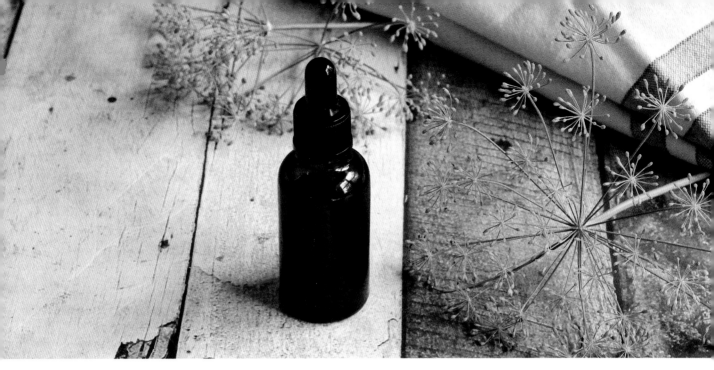

 # DILL MASSAGE OIL FOR COLICKY BABIES

There is hardly a more frustrating moment as a parent than when your baby has a crampy, irritable stomach and they are virtually inconsolable. Their wails of pain are matched only by our agony over not being able to help much. Dill is a classic remedy for colicky babies and one that works with astonishing consistency. Applied as a massage oil and followed by skin-to-skin contact, this dill will help to calm poor fussy infants and tired, flustered parents alike.

While this remedy is specifically geared for babies, there is no reason why it can't be used for older children and adults.

YIELD: approximately 4+ ounces (120 ml)

INGREDIENTS

4 oz (120 ml) sweet almond oil

2 tbsp (20 g) dried dill seeds and/or dried dill leaf

INSTRUCTIONS

In a jar with a tight-fitting lid, infuse the sweet almond oil with dill using any of the infusion methods mentioned on page 12. After the infusion is complete, strain the oil through two layers of flour sack cloth into a liquid measuring cup, wringing and squeezing to extract all the oil. Pour into a 4-ounce (120-ml) dropper bottle.

To use, apply several drops to a bare baby belly and massage into the tummy in a clockwise circular motion, using gentle strokes and warm hands. After the massage, it is best to have skin-to-skin contact with the baby to keep the belly warm until the colic passes. Use within 1 year.

FENNEL

OTHER COMMON NAMES: sow/hog fennel, sulphur wort, marsh parsley, chucklusa

LATIN NAME: *Foeniculum vulgare*

HERBAL ENERGETICS: warm/dry

THERAPEUTIC ACTIONS: antibacterial, antifungal, antihirsutism, anti-inflammatory, antioxidant, antithrombotic, antitussive, carminative, diuretic, expectorant, galactagogue, hepatic, hypoglycemic, sialagogue

PARTS USED: seed, (fronds, bulb, pollen edible)

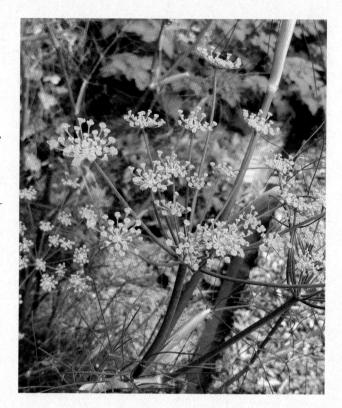

HERBAL MONOGRAPH

Fennel was an "acquired" taste for me. In fact, I generally disliked anything with anise-y, licorice-y notes. It wasn't until my palate "matured" that I grew to appreciate fennel for its culinary attributes. Which gave me a chance to experience its medicinal attributes without even knowing it. Something about eating a meal infused with fennel made me feel light and healthy, without any lingering sense of slow digestion or upset stomach. Fennel makes the case for food as medicine—in a really refreshing way!

Fennel has a truly diverse array of therapeutic actions, chief among them being its incredible soothing effects on the digestive system. Fennel provides fast-acting relief from bloating and gas the likes of which makes one want to unbutton one's pants. This is especially true for those that experience more eruptive, flatulent emissions. Fennel is one of the gentlest herbs to help with infant colic, and is often a favored ingredient in "gripe water." This herb also stimulates the flow of saliva, increasing one's appetite and promoting digestive action. It is perfect for those with weak, atonic stomachs that are slow to process a meal. Additionally, fennel helps to moderate post-meal spikes in blood sugar resulting in post-meal malaise—making it the perfect flavor to add to a midday meal to prevent the dreaded post-lunch slump.

Fennel is an undervalued herb for the respiratory system. It best serves the individual with a tight, hacking spasmodic cough that simply won't loosen its grip. Fennel soothes inflamed airways and calms the irritation that perpetuates the persistent, unrelenting reflex to cough, making it an ideal herbal ally for whooping cough and bronchitis. Studies also show that fennel can have a positive effect on those suffering from type IV allergic reactions (delayed hypersensitivity to triggering substances).

As an antioxidant and a hepatic herb, fennel has a protective effect on the liver. It can also help to stimulate the flow of breast milk. Some studies have even indicated that the constituents in fennel have some anticlotting action, warranting further study of this herb for anticoagulant therapies.

BEST PREPARATIONS: Fennel seeds make flavorful teas, infusions and tinctures and can even be chewed on for immediate gas relief and freshened breath. Honey infused with fennel seeds is very soothing for respiratory complaints.

Fennel is a tasty vegetable that lends itself to many types of meals. The seeds and fronds can be used to infuse a subtle anise flavor that is especially nice with chicken or fish. The bulb can be grilled for a really interesting flavor and texture or shaved very thin and paired with apples and cabbage for an amazing slaw. Even fennel pollen is now being used for culinary purposes.

HERBAL SUBSTITUTES: Dill (*Anethum graveolens*): carminative | wild cherry bark (*Prunus serotina*): antitussive

SAFETY AND PRECAUTIONS

Do not use if you are taking anticoagulant therapies. If you are pregnant, nursing or taking prescription medication, please consult your physician before taking this or any other herb. Fennel as used for food is considered safe.

LOOK-ALIKES: Dill (*Anethum graveolens*)

IDENTIFY & GROW

TYPE OF PLANT: Perennial

HABITAT: Fennel prefers sunny locations, with well-drained soils

HEIGHT: 4–5' (1–1.5 m)

LEAF: Threadlike green fronds with characteristic "anise-y" scent

STEM: Hollow stem arising from a bulb-like base

FLOWER: Petite stems bearing small sprays of tiny yellow flowers top singular stems to form an open umbel

SEED: Light green seeds mature in late summer.

GROWING INFORMATION: Soak seeds before planting directly in a sunny location. Water frequently through germination and establishment. Plant well away from dill to prevent cross-pollination and oddly flavored seeds. Fennel should be planted at the back of borders due to its height. Fennel has a slightly allopathic effect and may discourage other nearby plantings.

FORAGE OR GROW? Wild fennel can be found in coastal and riverside areas, but it is largely a cultivated botanical. Fennel grows easily from seed, making it appropriate for the home garden if given a designated area.

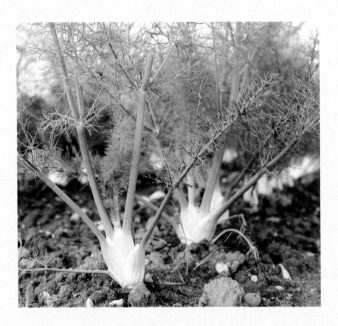

BEST HARVEST PRACTICES

LEAF/FROND HARVEST WINDOW: Summer

BULB HARVEST WINDOW: Summer

SEED HARVEST WINDOW: Late summer to early fall

Fennel fronds can be harvested at any time while the herb is fresh and green. Seeds can be left to mature on the flower head until it adequately dries. When seeds are brown and dry, cover each seed head with a paper bag, snip the stalk and shake the flower head vigorously into the bag.

TIP: Culinary and medicinal herbs are often exceptionally good companion plants for the home garden. This is not the case with fennel! This tasty bulb with its wonderfully medicinal seeds actually inhibits the growth and development of surrounding plants. To include this useful medicinal in your garden, consider growing it in a container or at least 3–5 feet (1–1.5 m) away from other herbs, fruits and vegetables.

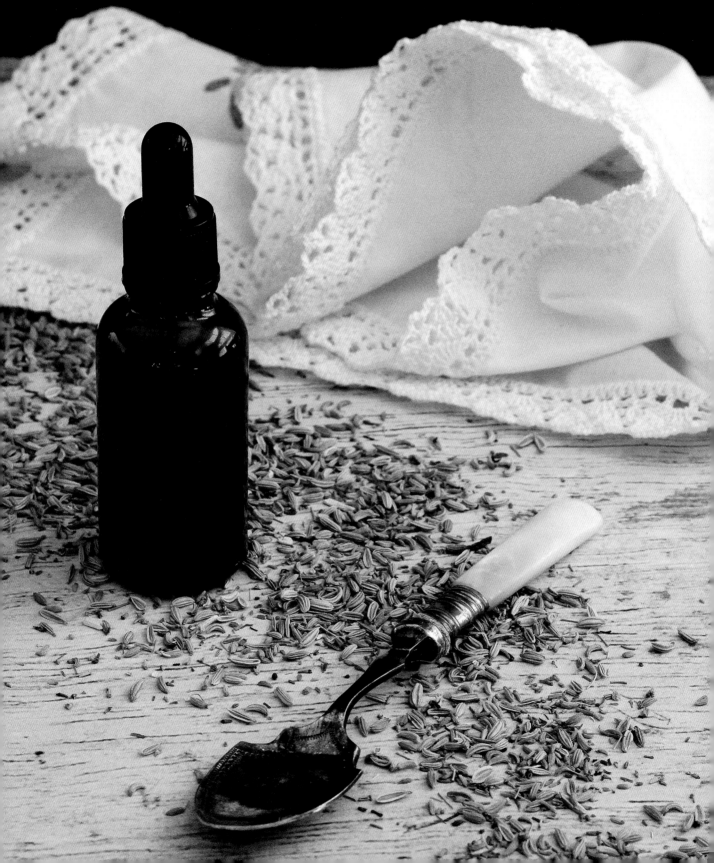

FENNEL GRIPE WATER FOR FUSSY BABIES & TUMMY-TROUBLED TODDLERS

My older children were largely unfazed by gassy or troubled tummies, but when my littlest one arrived I got my first taste of colic. Although we were lucky in that she had short colicky bouts, I felt nothing but sheer frustration about my inability to soothe her upset. Gripe water became a real saving grace during those early months—saving her from pain and me from sleepless nights.

Fennel soothes gassy tummies and irritable infant bowels. It even quells spasmodic hiccups. This blend is preserved with vegetable glycerin, which adds sweetness. This gripe water should be refrigerated between uses and a fresh batch made every 7 to 10 days to ensure freshness.

YIELD: about 4 ounces (120 ml)

INFANT'S DOSE, AGES 0-6 MONTHS: 1–5 drops as needed

INFANT'S DOSE, AGES 6-12 MONTHS: 10–15 drops, as needed

CHILD'S DOSE, AGES 12 MONTHS TO 6 YEARS: 1–2 teaspoons (5–10 ml), as needed

ADULT DOSE: 1 tablespoon (15 ml), as needed

INGREDIENTS

1 tbsp (10 g) dried fennel seeds

½ cup (120 ml) water

1 tbsp (15 ml) organic vegetable glycerin

INSTRUCTIONS

Combine the fennel with water just off the boil. Infuse for 20 minutes. Strain the fennel tea into a small liquid measuring cup. Add the vegetable glycerin to the cooled and strained fennel infusion.

Pour into two 2-ounce (60-ml) amber glass dropper bottles. Use within 10 days.

CORN SILK

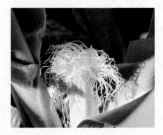

OTHER COMMON NAMES: corn tassel

LATIN NAME: *Zea mays*

HERBAL ENERGETICS: cool/neutral

THERAPEUTIC ACTIONS: anti-inflammatory, antimicrobial, antioxidant, antispasmodic, astringent, cholagogue, demulcent, diuretic, hypoglycemic, hypolipidemic, hypotensive

PARTS USED: corn silks

HERBAL MONOGRAPH

Corn on the cob is the ubiquitous late summer treat. Boiled or grilled and slathered with butter and seasonings, fresh corn is hard to resist—even for those of us who disdain food that gets caught in our teeth. Corn is a harvest tradition as much as it is a food, but corn as medicine is hardly on anybody's radar. Which is altogether unfortunate, as corn silks are one of the most effective and gentle herbs to address complaints of the genito-urinary system.

Corn silks offer lasting relief to a variety of urinary complaints such as pelvic pressure, incontinence, frequent urge to urinate with low output and burning with urination. It is part of the many herbal protocols for cystitis and interstitial cystitis, as well as urinary tract infections. Corn silks are very useful to ease the pain and encourage the dissolution of kidney stones. Corn silk is often suggested for addressing concerns of an enlarged prostate in men, and, in a 2017 study, it was shown to improve symptoms of benign prostatic hyperplasia. This botanical is a strong antioxidant that helps to protect the kidneys and liver from oxidative damage caused by certain medications and drug use.

The diuretic actions of corn silks have implications beyond that of the immediate renal system. This herb is often used to help flush uric acid from the body to the benefit of gout sufferers. The removal of excessive fluids also aids those with puffy, baggy eyes, rheumatoid arthritis and high blood pressure.

Corn silks also help to increase and thin bile, which greatly reduces digestive upset after eating a meal high in fats. It also helps to prevent post-meal crashes in blood glucose levels.

BEST PREPARATIONS: Fresh or dried corn silks can be prepared as a tea or infusion. Tinctures should be used with fresh herb when at all possible.

HERBAL SUBSTITUTES: Cleavers (*Galium aparine*): diuretic

SAFETY AND PRECAUTIONS

Corn silks are considered safe while pregnant and for minor kidney complaints. Always consult with a physician about acute complaints. Please consult with a physician if you are taking prescription medication.

LOOK-ALIKES: None

IDENTIFY & GROW

TYPE OF PLANT: Annual

HABITAT: Corn prefers full sun. Plant in fertile, deep soils, and water frequently.

HEIGHT: 8–12' (2.5–3.5 m)

LEAF: Light green leaves clasp the central stalk. Leaves have prominent ridges.

FLOWER: Silks are the female part of the corn flower that is hidden inside the maturing husk. Depending on the variety, these threadlike plumes are observed in shades of beige to bright pink when mature.

GROWING INFORMATION: Sow corn kernels directly into well-worked soil after all danger of frost has passed. Water frequently throughout germination and the growing season. Corn is a heavy feeder requiring amendment where soils are poor. Protect from heavy wind when possible

FORAGE OR GROW? While corn may volunteer the next year, it is unlikely to be the same variety as the previous year, as this botanical hybridizes readily. Plant from seed to ensure you have a desirable variety so that you may enjoy the corn as well as the silks.

BEST HARVEST PRACTICES

CORNSILK HARVEST WINDOW: Summer to early fall

Corn silks can be trimmed from the husk as the corn is almost mature, but the silks have not yet browned. When shucking corn, you can use the silks inside the husk as well, trimming away dried and browned areas.

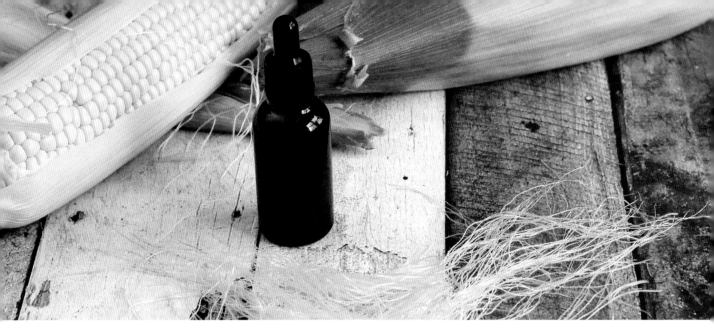

CORN SILK TINCTURE FOR URINARY, PROSTATE AND PELVIC FLOOR HEALTH

You've been throwing away one of nature's most effective and gentle medicines every summer and early fall. Every time you shuck your ears of corn and drop the husks and silks into the compost, you are discarding one of the best remedies for the urinary tract, prostate and pelvic areas! So, instead of tossing those sticky corn silks, next time toss them into a jar of spirits!

YIELD: 1 pint (480 ml)

ADULT DOSE: 3–5 droppers full (4.5–7.5 ml), 3 times daily

CHILD'S DOSE, AGES 6-12: 1–3 droppers full (1.5–4.5 ml), 3 times daily

NOT RECOMMENDED FOR CHILDREN UNDER THE AGE OF 6:
If there is poor urine output or painful urination in small children, please consult your physician.

INGREDIENTS

2 cups (480 ml) 80 proof spirits (vodka recommended)

1 cup (30 g) corn silks, packed

INSTRUCTIONS

Place the spirits and corn silks in a jar with a tight-fitting lid. Infuse for a minimum of 6 weeks, shaking daily. After the tincture is adequately infused, strain through two layers of flour sack cloth into a liquid measuring cup. Pour into 1- or 2-ounce (30- or 60-ml) amber glass dropper bottles or a pint-sized (480-ml) amber glass master bottle for dispensing. Use within 1 year.

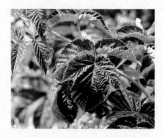

RASPBERRY LEAF

OTHER COMMON NAMES: brambleberry

LATIN NAME: *Rubus idaeus, R. occidentalis, R. strigosus*

HERBAL ENERGETICS: cool/dry

THERAPEUTIC ACTIONS: anti-inflammatory, astringent, diaphoretic, digestive, diuretic, laxative, nutritive, tonic

PARTS USED: leaf, root, fruit (edible)

HERBAL MONOGRAPH

Medicine is often no farther than the backyard garden or the farm down the road. While raspberries are the epitome of summery berry goodness, not many take notice of the brilliant raspberry leaf itself. While the sun-ripened ruby berries are surely dazzling and tempting in their own right, a good herbalist knows that the benefits of this botanical are not limited to its ripe fruit!

Red raspberry leaf is most closely associated with womb health. Red raspberry leaf teas are often suggested for late in a pregnancy to fortify and strengthen the uterus for the coming labor-some event. Some herbalists suggest its use earlier in a pregnancy to help prevent miscarriage and quell morning sickness, although there are some indications that it may be too stimulating to be appropriate at this fragile time. This botanical is also suggested for a lax, atonic uterus after birth and weepy postpartum bleeding. Beyond the window of imminent and post labor, raspberry leaf is indicated for excessive menstrual flow, delayed menses and a sense of heaviness about the abdomen.

Raspberry leaf is also a tonic for the urinary tract. It is well-suited for those suffering from an irritable bladder, incontinence and pelvic floor dysfunction as it helps to tone and support bladder tissues. It is also suggested for prostate health, helping to decrease urinary urges and increase flow. Raspberry leaves are also considered a laxative, contributing to lower-abdominal wellness.

BEST PREPARATIONS: Red raspberry leaves make a nice tea or infusion with slight fruity overtones. Leaves can be tinctured fresh. The root can be decocted with similar action to the leaf.

Raspberries are a prized summer treat, and they make the most delectable jams and jellies. For a simple, no-fuss summertime dessert, I love a few raspberries with fresh whipped cream and crumbled amaretti cookies!

HERBAL SUBSTITUTES: Blackberry (*Rubus* sp.): astringent

SAFETY AND PRECAUTIONS

Do not use until the final weeks of pregnancy. If you are pregnant, nursing or taking prescription medication, please contact your physician before using this or any other herb.

LOOK-ALIKES: Other *Rubus* species

IDENTIFY & GROW

⚘ **TYPE OF PLANT:** Perennial

⚘ **HABITAT:** Raspberries like full sun and deep, rich, well-drained soils.

⚘ **HEIGHT:** Trailing vine 8–10' (2–3 m) in length if left to grow unchecked.

⚘ **LEAF:** Pinnate, compound, serrated light green leaves arranged alternately on the vine

⚘ **STEM:** Vines covered in small thorn-like hairs

⚘ **FLOWER:** White five-petaled flowers appear early summer and are very attractive to pollinators.

⚘ **FRUIT:** Cone to dome-shaped fruit covered in fine hairs that pulls easily away from a white pithy center when ripe.

⚘ **GROWING INFORMATION:** Raspberries are best propagated by division. Plant in an area of full sun with well-amended soils, somewhat protected from the wind. Most varieties bear fruit in the second year (floracane). Each fall, prune woody stems to the ground and select for next year's fruit-bearing canes.

⚘ **FORAGE OR GROW?** There are some wild raspberries to be found, but these vines are best to grow.

BEST HARVEST PRACTICES

LEAF AND FRUIT HARVEST WINDOW: Summer

Leaves can be harvested throughout the growing season. Do not take too many leaves from one cane as it will reduce photosynthesis.

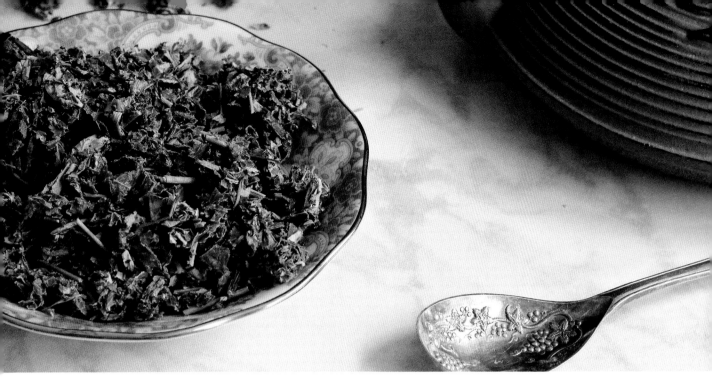

 # RASPBERRY LEAF TEA FOR IMPENDING LABOR

While it is a mixed bag of opinions about the safety of red raspberry early in a pregnancy, most herbalists and midwives agree that red raspberry used in the weeks leading up to delivery promotes a healthy progressive labor experience for mother and infant. With a green and fruity flavor, I find this a very sip-able simple tea, sweetened slightly with honey to taste.

This tea is also supportive for women trying to conceive in the 2 weeks prior to ovulation.

YIELD: 1 serving

ADULT DOSE: 2–3 cups (480–720 ml) of tea daily (after 35 weeks gestation)

INGREDIENTS

8–10 oz (240–300 ml) water just off the boil

1 tbsp (3 g) dried raspberry leaf

Raw, unfiltered honey, to taste (optional)

INSTRUCTIONS

Steep the red raspberry leaf in hot water for 5 to 7 minutes. Strain, and sweeten with honey to taste (if using). Use within 1 year.

TIP: With pregnancy, I prefer to keep formulas simple and gentle to help ensure the safety of mother and child.

PEPPERMINT

OTHER COMMON NAMES: yerba buena

LATIN NAME: *Mentha* x *piperita*

HERBAL ENERGETICS: warm/cool/dry

THERAPEUTIC ACTIONS: analgesic, anodyne, antiemetic, antifungal, anti-inflammatory, antioxidant, antispasmodic, astringent, cardiovascular, carminative, cholagogue, diaphoretic, diffusive, emmenagogue, expectorant, hepatic, insect repellant, nervine, stimulant

PARTS USED: aerial parts

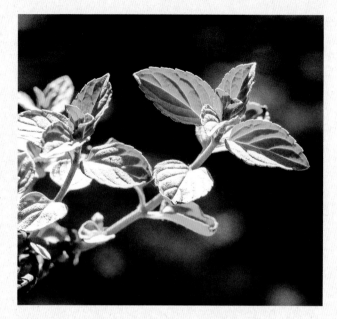

HERBAL MONOGRAPH

Peppermint is to the herbal world what vanilla is to desserts. So ubiquitous that it seems almost mundane. They say that familiarity breeds contempt—though I would suggest that familiarity breeds indifference. We lose sight of the value of peppermint (and vanilla, for that matter), because it is so accessible. But it is because of its accessibility that peppermint should receive so much praise. I have heard many wise herbalists suggest that while peppermint is not the cure for all that ails, it will certainly bring relief to almost any complaint. Simply put, peppermint offers something to everyone. Trust in its value.

I first came to know peppermint in its medicinal form in the oddest, yet most common of ways: as complimentary mints given out at restaurants at the end of meals. Those mint candies always seemed to take the edge off my childhood stomach upset. When I found my path as an herbalist, I hardly had to read the literature on peppermint to confirm its carminative effects. Peppermint calmed. That much I knew. Peppermint has long been used for digestive upsets such as nausea, motion sickness, indigestion and bloating. More recent studies suggest that enterically coated peppermint essential oil capsules may be even more effective at combatting the complaint of irritable bowel syndrome with diarrhea. Similarly, it is very soothing for all matters of menstrual pain and pelvic/lower back cramping.

Peppermint is also associated with pain relief and is most especially effective for tension headaches. Diluted essential oil applied to the temples, or a cool compress of peppermint infusion draping the forehead can bring relief to tired, overworked brains and computer-strained eyes. Peppermint can also soothe painful, rheumatic joints and strained muscles.

Peppermint is a wonderful herb for congestion and upper respiratory complaints. As a stimulating and diffusive herb, it helps the "breakup" of stubborn congestion and drains boggy nasal sinuses. It also helps to reduce fever and heat associated with mild infections. Tea or a facial steam with peppermint is often all that it takes to open up airways and refresh the senses.

Peppermint, as well as other members of the mint family, have complicated herbal energetics. Upon tasting peppermint, one is greeted with an immediate surge of heat that is very quickly replaced by a profound and lasting cooling. As such, peppermint is ideal for cooling the body from heat and exertion. Peppermint is ideally suited for summer beverages after a hard afternoon of yard work.

BEST PREPARATIONS: Peppermint teas and infusions are most enjoyable, and the herb is often used as an adjunct to bitter herbs to increase palatability. Base oils can be infused with this aromatic herb for a cooling and aromatic massage oil. Fresh peppermint can be tinctured with a very tasty outcome. Essential oils can be diluted for topical application. Use internally in the form of enterically coated capsules under the guidance of a qualified aromatherapy professional only. Poultices of fresh peppermint can be applied to sore teeth and gums.

Peppermint is a delightful culinary herb. I love it chopped finely with parsley and mixed into plain Greek yogurt or wheat berries. It can be muddled into the bottom of a glass for minty cocktails and sparkling water. Mint is an herb frequently used in Mediterranean and Middle Eastern cuisine, where it lends a bright pop of flavor to the palate.

HERBAL SUBSTITUTES: Spearmint (*Mentha spicata*)

SAFETY AND PRECAUTIONS
Do not used peppermint if you suffer from GERD, as it relaxes the lower esophageal sphincter. If you are pregnant, nursing or taking prescription medication, please consult your physician before taking this or any other herb.

LOOK-ALIKES: Other *Mentha* species

IDENTIFY & GROW

🌼 **TYPE OF PLANT:** Perennial

🌼 **HABITAT:** Peppermint prefers full sun to light shade and likes fairly rich, somewhat moist soils.

🌼 **HEIGHT:** 12–18" (30–45 cm)

🌼 **LEAF:** Deeply veined opposite, ovoid, green leaves with serrated edges. New growth is often somewhat purple in color. Characteristically fragrant.

🌼 **STEM:** Square; may be purple in areas

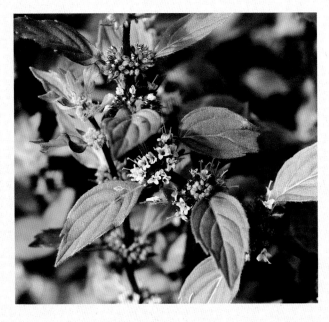

🌼 **FLOWER:** White to lilac flowers appear in whorls atop stems early to mid-summer

🌼 **GROWING INFORMATION:** Peppermint grows easily from cuttings. Or peppermint seeds can be started indoors 6 to 8 weeks before the last frost or sown directly in the garden after frost has passed. Peppermint can be quite aggressive so give it plenty of room to spread or consider planting in a container.

🌼 **FORAGE OR GROW?** There is an abundance of wild and feral mints with similar therapeutic actions throughout most temperate climates. It may be difficult to determine exact species as mints hybridize readily. If you are particularly set on peppermint, I would consider growing it.

BEST HARVEST PRACTICES
LEAF AND FLOWERING TOP PEAK HARVEST WINDOW: Mid-summer

Peppermint is at its peak when in flower. Cut within about 6 inches (15 cm) of the soil line to encourage new growth.

JADE GODDESS TEA

Soothing, cooling and relaxing—that is what summer evenings should be about. Make this minty herbal tea blend by the gallon and store in the refrigerator for the most refreshing tea when the temperature requires multiple fans and absolutely no body part touching another. This tea will cool you from head to toe when the summer sun makes even your elbows sweat! It is also a soothing tea that I love to sip while on a car ride to prevent motion sickness or when a general upset tummy is experienced!

For a lighter flavor, steep sprigs of these fresh herbs in cold water for a refreshing thirst quencher.

YIELD: 4 cups (100 g) dried tea blend

INGREDIENTS

2 cups (50 g) dried peppermint

1 cup (25 g) dried lemon balm

1 cup (25 g) dried catmint

INSTRUCTIONS

Combine the dried herbs, and store in a tight-lidded jar in a cool, dry place.

To make tea, steep ½ to 1 cup (13 to 25 g) of the herbal mixture in 4 cups (960 ml) of water just off the boil for at least 20 minutes for a strong infusion. Strain the infusion through a fine-mesh sieve into a gallon-sized (4-L) beverage container. Fill the container with ice and water until full. Keep chilled. Serve with a fresh sprig of mint and a slice of lemon, if you are feeling fancy. Use within 1 year.

Drink as desired; safe for children.

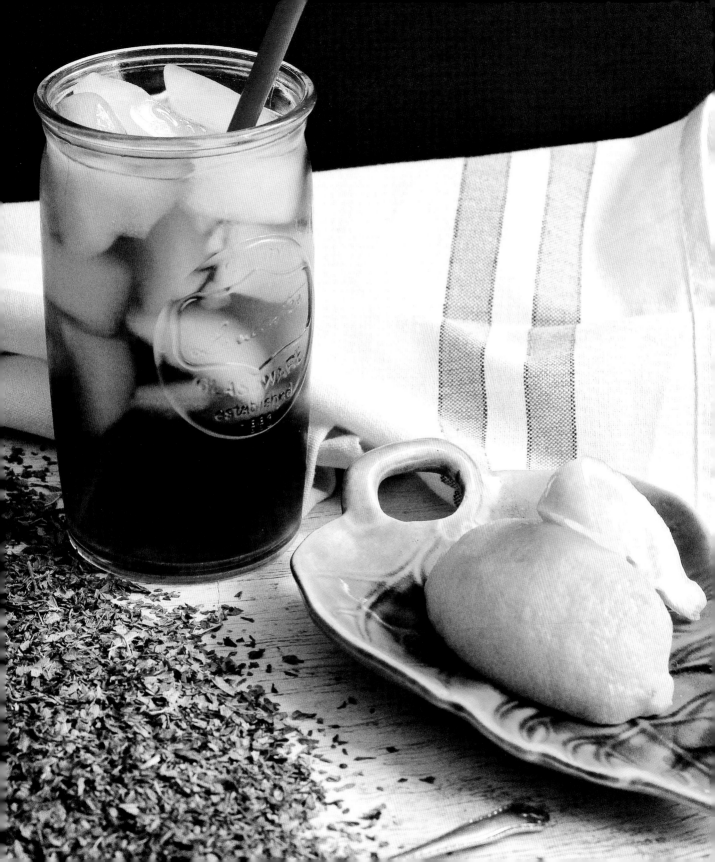

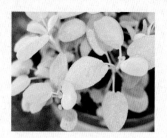

SAGE

OTHER COMMON NAMES: salvia, sarubia

LATIN NAME: *Salvia officinalis*

HERBAL ENERGETICS: cool/dry

THERAPEUTIC ACTIONS: anti-inflammatory, antimicrobial, antiseptic, antispasmodic, astringent, carminative, diaphoretic, diuretic, emmenagogue, hepatic, nervine

PARTS USED: leaves

HERBAL MONOGRAPH

Sage is the scent of holiday birds and fall meals. It is a comforting fragrance and a tasty herb. It is also a wonderfully medicinal herb with a (gravy) boatload of therapeutic actions.

Sage is a soothing anti-inflammatory herb with a particular affinity for complaints of the mouth. This herb is calming to redness and inflammation about the throat and tonsils. Sage is often recommended for laryngitis, tonsillitis and allergic asthma. It is also an ideal choice of medicinal herb for spongy bleeding gums, mouth ulcers and abscesses.

Sage is my favorite herb to turn to when there are complaints of heat. For menopausal women suffering from hot flashes, sage offers unparcelled moderation of those intense episodes of volcanic heat. It is also an herb that I offer those going through alcohol withdrawal to help curb night sweats. As a nervine herb, sage also benefits memory and cognition.

Perhaps it should come as no surprise that an herb that we so commonly associate with big, hearty meals is also an outstanding digestive herb. Sage is a choice herb to address upset stomach, gas and bloating. Sage's dry energetics make it an excellent remedy for those who have excessive mucus in the digestive tract, such as experienced during a head cold or sinus infection. It is well suited for those who tend to overeat (and overdrink) at a meal.

BEST PREPARATIONS: Sage makes a very savory tea or infusion. A cooled infusion with a pinch of sea salt will make a very soothing gargle for sore throat complaints. Sage-infused honey is an excellent remedy for small children and fussier adults when the flavor of more medicinal syrups is found objectionable. A tincture made from fresh sage is most ideal for cooling and nervine benefits.

Sage is a popular culinary herb that pairs well with poultry, fowl and sweet winter squash. One of my favorite, if unusual, uses of sage is to combine it with wild blackberries in a shrub (a traditional sweetened, flavored vinegar-based beverage) that I mix with sparkling water for a cooling summery drink.

HERBAL SUBSTITUTES: Bee balm (*Monarda* sp.): expectorant | peppermint (*Mentha* x *piperita*): diaphoretic

SAFETY AND PRECAUTIONS

Sage is safe when used in quantities normal in food. If you are pregnant, nursing or taking prescription medication, please consult your physician before using this or any other herb.

LOOK-ALIKES: Lamb's ear (*Salvia byzantina*), clary sage (*Salvia sclarea*)

IDENTIFY & GROW

TYPE OF PLANT: Perennial

HABITAT: Sage prefers full sun to light shade in sandy, well-drained soils.

HEIGHT: 12–24" (30–60 cm)

LEAF: Pale green or variegated leaves are arranged opposite. Leaves have a velvety texture due to the presence of very fine hairs called trichomes.

STEM: New growth starts green but becomes woody as the plant matures.

FLOWER: Lilac, lipped flowers appear in whorls atop stems in early summer.

GROWING INFORMATION: Sage is most easily propagated from cuttings. Plant sage starts in a sunny location with well-drained soil. Resist the urge to fertilize the plant, as leaner soils will promote a greater amount of volatile oil in the leaves.

FORAGE OR GROW? Sage may be difficult to find in the wild, making this an appropriate herb to grow.

BEST HARVEST PRACTICES

HARVEST WINDOW: Sage can be harvested during the whole growing season. Unlike many herbs, the amount of volatile oil actually increases as the leaves grow larger after flowering.

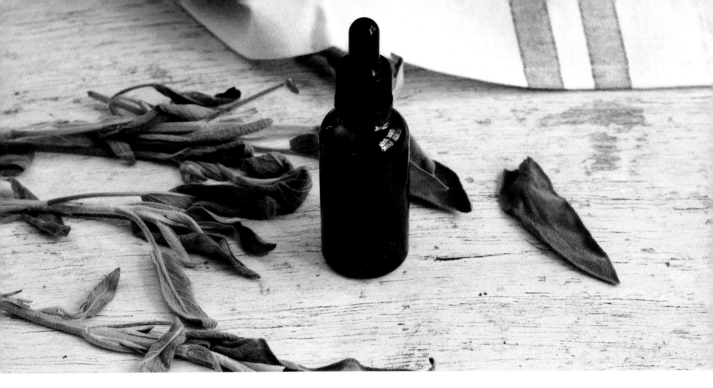

SUPER DUTY SAGE TINCTURE FOR HOT CONDITIONS

Sage is my heavy lifter. Not only does it serve as the flavor backbone for the holiday bird, but it is a medicinal superhero as well. Sage is best suited for those who experience hot conditions. It is the first herb that I reach for when there are complaints of hot flashes and night sweats, and it is an excellent remedy to tight, hot throats, especially when used as a gargle in salt water.

YIELD: 1 pint (480 ml)

ADULT DOSE: 1–3 droppers full (1.5–4.5 ml), 3 times daily

CHILD'S DOSE, AGES 6–12: ½–1 dropper full (0.75–1.5 ml), 3 times daily

GARGLE: Add 5–10 drops sage tincture to a small amount of water with a pinch of sea salt. Gargle for 10 to 15 seconds.

INGREDIENTS

2 cups (480 ml) 100 proof spirits (vodka recommended)

1½ cups (45 g) chopped fresh sage

INSTRUCTIONS

Combine the spirits and sage in a jar with a tight-fitting lid. Infuse for a minimum of 6 weeks, shaking daily. After the infusion is complete, strain through two layers of flour sack cloth into a liquid measuring cup. Pour into 1- or 2-ounce (30- or 60-ml) amber glass dropper bottles or into a pint-sized (480-ml) amber glass master bottle for dispensing. Use within 1 year.

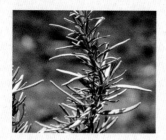

ROSEMARY

OTHER COMMON NAMES: compass weed, dew of the sea

LATIN NAME: *Rosmarinus officinalis*

HERBAL ENERGETICS: warm/dry

THERAPEUTIC ACTIONS: anti-inflammatory, antimicrobial, antioxidant, cardiovascular, carminative, expectorant, hepatic, nervine, stimulant

PARTS USED: aboveground parts

HERBAL MONOGRAPH

My father has always had a knack for rosemary. In one of his many gardens, he grew beds of rosemary as tall as a man and twice as wide. They say that rosemary is for remembrance—and my memories of rosemary are vivid indeed.

Rosemary is a warming, stimulating herb that helps to raise low blood pressure and increase circulation, helping those with cool fingers and toes and generally cold constitutions. With this invigorating action, rosemary benefits the brain and has long been noted to enhance memory. Rosemary has been used as a remedy for senility, and recent studies have indicated that rosemary appears to increase recollection, improve cognition and promote memory recall—implications for students and the elderly alike.

Rosemary is also both stimulating and protective for the skin and hair. Rosemary is a valuable source of antioxidants which neutralize the free radicals that damage and age the skin. Rosemary-based skincare products promote a rosy, refreshed complexion and reduce visible signs of aging. This herb is also suggested for thinning hair and premature balding, stimulating the scalp and encouraging voluminous locks. Brunette and black-haired beauties can rinse their hair with rosemary infusions to attain luster and shine.

Rosemary was also suggested as one of the possible "thieves herbs" associated with the prevention of Black Plague transmission, and there is mounting evidence to support its uses as an antimicrobial agent. Rosemary is ideally used when one is plagued by a weepy, running nose and thick, chesty cough that produces as lot of sputum. Upset stomach and nausea caused by sinus drainage is also greatly relieved by rosemary use. This herb also helps to stimulate efficient digestion, and it is perfect for those that feel leaden and cold after a meal.

BEST PREPARATIONS: Rosemary produces wonderfully warming teas and infusions, and makes a lovely pine-flavored tincture as well. Rosemary infuses beautifully in honey for respiratory complaints. Base oils infused with rosemary are great for massage and skin protection creams. Distilled vinegar infused with rosemary makes a fantastic hair rinse.

HERBAL SUBSTITUTES: Thyme (*Thymus officinalis*): respiratory | self heal (*Prunella vulgaris*): antioxidant

SAFETY AND PRECAUTIONS

Rosemary is safe in amounts used in food. Avoid using rosemary medicinally if you suffer from high blood pressure. If you are pregnant, nursing or taking prescription medication, please consult your physician before taking this or any other herb.

LOOK-ALIKES: Dog fennel (*Eupatorium capillifolium*)

IDENTIFY & GROW

🌸 TYPE OF PLANT: Perennial

🌸 HABITAT: Rosemary likes full sun and relatively dry, well-drained soils.

🌸 HEIGHT: 3–5' (1–1.5 m); low-growing, trailing cultivars of rosemary are common

🌸 LEAF: Fragrant, needle-like, evergreen leaves arrange opposite in a woody stem

🌸 STEM: Flexible, new green growth matures to a woody stem.

🌸 FLOWER: Most rosemary flowers are blue, although white, pink and lilac flowers have been observed. Flowers appear early to mid-summer.

🌸 GROWING INFORMATION: Rosemary is best propagated by cutting. Plant starts in a sunny location with sandy and well-drained soils.

🌸 FORAGE OR GROW? Wild rosemary can be found around the Mediterranean and areas in which it has naturalized, but this is an easy herb for most folks to grow.

BEST HARVEST PRACTICES
ABOVEGROUND PARTS HARVEST WINDOW: Summer

Rosemary has the best aromatic, medicinal profile if harvested at the time of flowering, although it can be harvested at virtually any time of year.

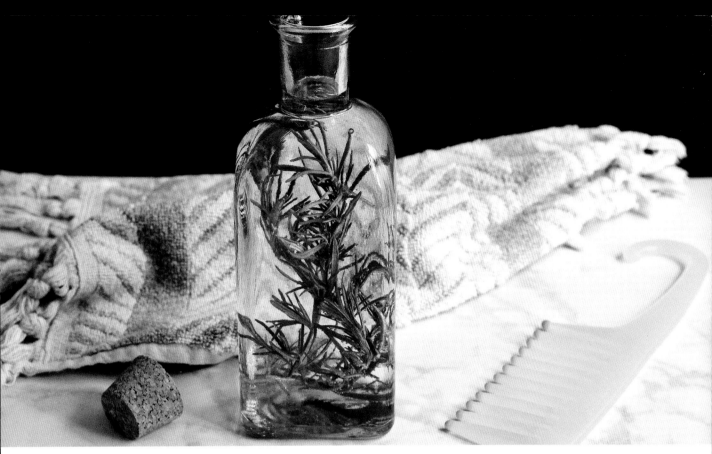

 # ROSEMARY HAIR RINSE FOR SHINY, LUSTROUS LOCKS

Rosemary has always been touted for its ability to bring shine and luster to dark locks. It also soothes itchy, flaky scalps and stimulates the hair follicle. Vinegar is a surprising conditioner and helps to detangle long hair. Combined, rosemary and vinegar make an excellent hair rinse after shampoo! This rinse is excellent for "no-'pooers" and those using baking soda to wash their hair.

While this recipe is ideal for those with darker hair, the recipe can easily be adapted with other herbs. Blondes will like the shine from chamomile, and redheads will dazzle with hibiscus roselles used in place of the rosemary.

YIELD: 1 pint (480 ml)

INGREDIENTS

1 cup (30 g) chopped fresh rosemary

2 cups (480 ml) distilled white vinegar

INSTRUCTIONS

Combine the rosemary and vinegar in a jar with a tight-fitting lid. Slip a disc of parchment paper over the jar if using a metal lid. Infuse for 2 weeks, then strain through a fine-mesh sieve into a liquid measuring cup. Pour into a plastic "squeeze bottle" to use in the shower (safer than glass).

After shampooing, pour a small amount of the infused vinegar on your scalp working through to the ends of hair. Leave in your hair for 2 to 3 minutes, then rinse with lukewarm water. Use within 1 year.

TOOLS OF A WELL-PREPARED HERBALIST

Herbalism doesn't require a lot of special equipment. However, there are a few tools that will make your tasks in the garden, out foraging and in the apothecary kitchen so much easier!

FOR GARDENING & FORAGING

APPROPRIATE FOOTWEAR: Different seasons and conditions require different footwear. For your comfort and safety, make sure you have the right footwear for the job.

BACKPACK OR CROSSBODY HARVESTING BAG: Choose a sturdy bag that fits your body shape well and distributes weight evenly. I like ones with a few extra pockets that I can stick my tools into.

BASKET(S): While the novelty of a basket might seem cliché, baskets are especially great for plant matter that you don't want bruised when shoved into a bag.

HORI HORI KNIFE OR POCKET KNIFE: A decent blade will allow you to do some trimming on the spot, often making for a more efficient harvest to pack out of the garden or woods.

KITCHEN SHEARS OR TRIMMERS: A smaller pair of kitchen or garden scissors make fast work of leaf and flower trimming on herbaceous, green growth.

PRUNING SHEARS: A good sturdy pair of pruning shears may make the task of trimming through woody stems and branches much easier when necessary.

REUSABLE MESH BAGS: These are great for leaves, roots and mushrooms, things that may be moist that you do not want to degrade due to humidity.

STURDY GLOVES: A good pair of leather gloves, or woven gloves with rubberized palms and fingers are invaluable and save you from pokey thorns and pricks. Nitrile or latex gloves may be desired for harvesting resinous materials.

ZIP CLOSURE BAGS: These are important for more resinous material such as cottonwood buds.

IN THE APOTHECARY KITCHEN

AMBER GLASS BOTTLES AND DROPPERS: Most liquid remedies benefit from the use of dark glass to minimize oxidation due to UV exposure.

DEDICATED SPATULAS, SPOONS, DRY AND LIQUID MEASURING CUPS AND SPOONS: Keep a set of these tools dedicated solely to your apothecary to prevent your next batch of cookies from tasting like last week's lotion.

DEHYDRATOR: For herbs that need to be dried quickly in low heat, such as cleavers, I highly recommend a dehydrator with an adjustable temperature setting and a fan.

DRYING SCREENS: Drying screens are perfect for drying flowers such as calendula and chamomile.

FINE-MESH SIEVE: Combined with flour sack cloths, a fine-mesh sieve is an excellent tool for making sure your remedy is grit free.

FLOUR SACK CLOTHS: While some folks may suggest straining preparations through cheesecloth or butter muslin, I prefer the size and weave of flour sack cloths for my herbal preparations.

FUNNEL(S): From canning jar funnels to tiny ones to fill half-ounce (14-ml) containers, a good supply of funnels makes for tidy packaging of finished remedies.

HEATPROOF GLASS BOWL OR DOUBLE BOILER: A dedicated bowl or double boiler makes salve making a breeze.

JARS: In a move that is likely to cause my husband's eyes to roll, there is no such thing as too many jars. From tiny jelly jars to gallon-sized (4-L) behemoths, you will likely find uses for every shape and size for the storage and preparation of your remedies.

KITCHEN SCALE: A small digital kitchen scale will give you precise measurements. This is particularly important for soapmaking as noted with the cedar soap on page 36.

RIMMED BAKING SHEETS: I prefer to dry woody roots on a baking sheet in an oven set to its lowest setting.

SLOW COOKER: I have two dedicated slow cookers—one mini and one regular size—that I use for rapid infusions and soap making.

TEA STRAINER OR FRENCH PRESS: Since I have little patience or the time it takes to fill individual tea bags, I like to have a French press and a few types of tea strainers on hand for my teas and infusions.

HERBAL ENERGETICS GLOSSARY

ALTERATIVE: Often referred to as "blood purifiers"; supports detoxification and elimination

ANALGESIC: Reduce perception of pain

ANODYNE: Pain reliever

ANTACID: Reduces stomach acidity

ANTHELMINTIC: Aids in the removal of intestinal parasites

ANTIBACTERIAL: Slows or halts the growth of bacteria

ANTIEMETIC: Helps prevent nausea and vomiting

ANTIHIRSUTISM: Suppresses excessive hair growth

ANTIHISTAMINE: Blocks the action of histamine; decreases allergenic response

ANTI-INFLAMMATORY: Decreases inflammation

ANTIMICROBIAL: Slows or halts microbial (bacterial, fungal and viral) growth

ANTINEOPLASTIC: Inhibits or halts the growth of a tumor

ANTI-OBTRUSANT: Draw out an irritant, such as a sliver or stinger, from tissues

ANTIOXIDANT: Prevents oxidative damage

ANTIPARASITIC: Slows or kills internal parasites

ANTIPERSPIRANT: Reduces perspiration

ANTI-PROLIFERATIVE: Reduces cellular growth

ANTI-RHEUMATIC: Helps to relieve discomfort due to rheumatism

ANTISEPTIC: Arrests decay of tissue due to microbes

ANTISPASMODIC: Relieves muscle cramping

ANTISPIROCHETAL: Slows or halts the bacteria growth of microbes specific to certain diseases such as Lyme

ANTITUSSIVE: Discourages spasmodic cough

ANTIVIRAL: Slows or halts the growth of viral infection

ANXIOLYTIC: Reduces anxiety

APERITIF: Stimulates appetite

ASTRINGENT: Tightens and tones tissue

BACTERIOSTATIC: Holds bacterial growth "in check"

CARDIOVASCULAR: Acts on the cardiovascular system

CARMINATIVE: Dispels gas and bloating

CELL PROLIFERANT: Encourages new cell growth

CHOLAGOGUE: Stimulates the cooling of gastric juices

DECONGESTANT: Reduces congestion, encourages sinus drainage

DEMULCENT: Slick, coating substance; emollient or mucilaginous

DIAPHORETIC: Encourages perspiration to cool

DIFFUSIVE: Stimulates; often profoundly warming

DIGESTIVE: Aids in various acts of digestion

DIURETIC: Encourages urination

EMMENAGOGUE: Acts on the female reproductive system

EMOLLIENT: Hydrating, creamy

EXPECTORANT: Stimulates productive cough; thins mucus

FEBRIFUGE: Reduces fever

GALACTOGOGUE: Increases the production of breast milk

HEPATIC: Acts on the liver; protects or aids in detoxification

HYPOGLYCEMIN: Suppresses elevated blood glucose levels

HYPOLIPEMIC: Aids in the reduction of lipids, such as cholesterol

HYPOTENSIVE: Reduces blood pressure

IMMUNE-MODULATING: Aids the immune system to issue appropriate immune response

LITHOTRYPTIC: Aids in the dissolution of "stones" in the urinary system

LYMPHATIC: Increases lymphatic flow and dissolves hardened nodes

NERVINE: Reduces anxiety and tension

NUTRITIVE: Vitamin- and mineral-rich herbs

ONEIROGEN: Thought to promote vivid and lucid dreams

PURGATIVE: Encourages vomiting

REFRIGERANT: Profoundly cooling herbs

RELAXANT: Relaxes

SEDATIVE: Calms; encourages sleep and restfulness

SIALAGOGUE: Increases saliva production

STIMULANT: Increases action

STYPTIC: Slows or arrests bleeding

TONIC: Tones organs

TROPHORESTORATIVE: Restores nutrients to support vitality

UTERINE STIMULANT: Stimulates uterine contraction

VASODILATOR: Dilates blood vessels

VERMIFUGE: Aids in the expulsion of internal parasites

VULNERARY: Speeds wound healing and closure

REFERENCES

Adhikari, Bhaskar Mani, Alina Bajracharya and Ashok K. Shrestha. "Comparison of nutritional properties of Stinging nettle (*Urtica dioica*) flour with wheat and barley flours." *Food Science & Nutrition* 4, no. 1 (2016): 119–124. doi:10.1002/fsn3.259.

Araújo, L. U., P. G. Reis, L. C. O. Barbosa, A. Grabe-Guimarães, V. C. F. Mosqueira, C. M. Carneiro, and N. M. Silva-Barcellos. "In vivo wound healing effects of *Symphytum officinale* L. leaves extract in different topical formulations." *Die Pharmazie—An International Journal of Pharmaceutical Sciences* 67, no. 4 (2012): 355–360.

Awaad, Amani A., Reham M. El-Meligy, Ghada M. Zain, Amal A. Safhi, Noura A. AL Qurain, Shekhah S. Almoqren, Yara M. Zain, Vidya D. Sesh Adri, and Fahad I. Al-Saikhan. "Experimental and clinical antihypertensive activity of *Matricaria chamomilla* extracts and their angiotensin-converting enzyme inhibitory activity." *Phytotherapy Research* (2018). doi:10.1002/ptr.6086.

Cheng, Xixi, Huafeng Wang, Jinlai Yang, Yingnan Cheng, Dan Wang, Fengrui Yang, Yan Li, et al. "Arctigenin protects against liver injury from acute hepatitis by suppressing immune cells in mice." *Biomedicine & Pharmacotherapy* 102 (2018): 464–471. doi:10.1016/j.biopha.2018.03.060.

Di Pierro, Francesco, Giuliana Rapacioli, Tarcisio Ferrara, and Stefano Togni. "Use of a standardized extract from *Echinacea angustifolia* (Polinacea) for the prevention of respiratory tract infections." *Altern Med Rev* 17, no. 1 (2012): 36–41.

Djemaa, Ferdaous Ghrab Ben, Khaled Bellassoued, Sami Zouari, Abdelfatteh El Feki, and Emna Ammar. "Antioxidant and wound healing activity of *Lavandula aspic* L. ointment." *Journal of Tissue Viability* 25, no. 4 (2016): 193–200. doi:10.1016/j.jtv.2016.10.002.

Dong, Pengzhi, Lanlan Pan, Xiting Zhang, Wenwen Zhang, Xue Wang, Meixiu Jiang, Yuanli Chen, et al. "Hawthorn (*Crataegus pinnatifida* Bunge) leave flavonoids attenuate atherosclerosis development in apoE knock-out mice." *Journal of Ethnopharmacology* 198 (2017): 479–488. doi:10.1016/j.jep.2017.01.040.

Farahani, Marzieh Sarbandi, Roodabeh Bahramsoltani, Mohammad Hosein Farzaei, Mohammad Abdollahi, and Roja Rahimi. "Plant-derived natural medicines for the management of depression: An overview of mechanisms of action." *Reviews in the Neurosciences* 26, no. 3 (2015): 305–321. doi:10.1515/revneuro-2014-0058.

Flora, Kenneth, Martin Hahn, Hugo Rosen, and Kent Benner. "Milk thistle (*Silybum marianum*) for the therapy of liver disease." *American Journal of Gastroenterology* 93, no. 2 (1998): 139.

Ghanim, Husam, Chang Ling Sia, Sanaa Abuaysheh, Kelly Korzeniewski, Priyanka Patnaik, Anuritha Marumganti, Ajay Chaudhuri, and Paresh Dandona. "An antiinflammatory and reactive oxygen species suppressive effects of an extract of *polygonum cuspidatum* containing resveratrol." *Molecular Endocrinology* 24, no. 7 (2010): 1498–1499. doi:10.1210/mend.24.7.9998.

Haghgoo, Roza, Majid Mehran, Elahe Afshari, Hamide Farajian Zadeh, and Motahare Ahmadvand. "Antibacterial effects of different concentrations of *Althaea officinalis* root extract versus 0.2% chlorhexidine and penicillin on Streptococcus mutans and Lactobacillus (in vitro)." *Journal of International Society of Preventive & Community Dentistry* 7, no. 4 (2017): 180. doi:10.4103/jispcd.JISPCD_150_17.

Ivanova, Diana, Oskan Tasinov, and Yoana Kiselova-Kaneva. "Improved lipid profile and increased serum antioxidant capacity in healthy volunteers after *Sambucus ebulus* L. fruit infusion consumption." *International Journal of Food Sciences and Nutrition* 65, no. 6 (2014): 740–744. doi:10.3109/09637486.2014.898256.

Jawad, Moutaz, R. Schoop, A. Suter, P. Klein, and Ronald Eccles. "Safety and efficacy profile of *Echinacea purpurea* to prevent common cold episodes: A randomized, double-blind, placebo-controlled trial." *Evidence-Based Complementary and Alternative Medicine* 2012 (2012). doi: 10.1155/2012/841315.

Jong, Miek C., Ulrike Ermuth, and Matthias Augustin. "Plant-based ointments versus usual care in the management of chronic skin diseases: A comparative analysis on outcome and safety." *Complementary Therapies in Medicine* 21, no. 5 (2013): 453–459. doi:10.1016/j.ctim.2013.07.002.

Karakaş, Fatma Pehlivan, Alper Karakaş, Çetin Boran, Arzu Uçar Türker, Funda Nuray Yalçin, and Erem Bilensoy. "The evaluation of topical administration of *Bellis perennis* fraction on circular excision wound healing in Wistar albino rats." *Pharmaceutical Biology* 50, no. 8 (2012): 1031–1037. doi:10.3109/13880209.2012.656200.

Kim, So Ra, Ae Wha Ha, Hyun Ji Choi, Sun Lim Kim, Hyeon Jung Kang, Myung Hwan Kim, and Woo Kyoung Kim. "Corn silk extract improves benign prostatic hyperplasia in experimental rat model." *Nutrition Research and Practice* 11, no. 5 (2017): 373–380. doi:10.4162/nrp.2017.11.5.373.

Lambert, Max Norman Tandrup, Catrine Bundgaard Thybo, Simon Lykkeboe, Lars Melholt Rasmussen, Xavier Frette, Lars Porskjær Christensen, and Per Bendix Jeppesen. "Combined bioavailable isoflavones and probiotics improve bone status and estrogen metabolism in postmenopausal osteopenic women: A randomized controlled trial." *American Journal of Clinical Nutrition* 106, no. 3 (2017): 909–920. doi:10.3945/ajcn.117.153353.

Martini, Silvia, Claudia D'Addario, Andrea Colacevich, Silvia Focardi, Francesca Borghini, Annalisa Santucci, Natale Figura, and Claudio Rossi. "Antimicrobial activity against *Helicobacter pylori* strains and antioxidant properties of blackberry leaves (*Rubus ulmifolius*) and isolated compounds." *International Journal of Antimicrobial Agents* 34, no. 1 (2009): 50–59. doi:10.1016/j.ijantimicag.2009.01.010.

Mueller, Monika, Stefanie Hobiger, and Alois Jungbauer. "Red clover extract: A source for substances that activate peroxisome proliferator-activated receptor α and ameliorate the cytokine secretion profile of lipopolysaccharide-stimulated macrophages." *Menopause* 17, no. 2 (2010): 379–387. doi:10.1097/gme.0b013e3181c94617.

Orchard, Ané, and Sandy van Vuuren. "Commercial essential oils as potential antimicrobials to treat skin diseases." *Evidence-Based Complementary and Alternative Medicine* 2017 (2017). doi:10.1155/2017/4517971.

Orhan, I. E. "Phytochemical and pharmacological activity profile of *Crataegus oxyacantha* L.(hawthorn)-A cardiotonic herb." *Current Medicinal Chemistry* (2016). doi:10.2174/0929867323666160919095519.

Ozalkaya, E., Z. Aslandogdu, A. Ozkoral, S. Topuoglu, and G. Karatekin. "Effect of a galactagogue herbal tea on breast milk production and prolactin secretion by mothers of preterm babies." *Nigerian Journal of Clinical Practice* (January 2018): 38–42. doi:10.4103/1119-3077.224788.

Pahlavan, Sara, Marziyeh Shalchi Tousi, Mahdi Ayyari, Abolfazl Alirezalu, Hassan Ansari, Tomo Saric, and Hossein Baharvand. "Effects of hawthorn (*Crataegus pentagyna*) leaf extract on electrophysiologic properties of cardiomyocytes derived from human cardiac arrhythmia–specific induced pluripotent stem cells." *FASEB Journal* 32, no. 3 (2017): 1440–1451. doi:10.1096/fj.201700494rr.

Powles, Trevor J., Anthony Howell, D. Gareth Evans, Eugene V. McCloskey, Sue Ashley, Rosemary Greenhalgh, Jenny Affen, Lesley Ann Flook, and Alwynne Tidy. "Red clover isoflavones are safe and well tolerated in women with a family history of breast cancer." *Menopause International* 14, no. 1 (2008): 6–12. doi:10.1258/mi.2007.007033.

Psotova, Jitka, Alena Svobodova, Hana Kolarova, and Daniela Walterova. "Photoprotective properties of *Prunella vulgaris* and rosmarinic acid on human keratinocytes." *Journal of Photochemistry and Photobiology B: Biology* 84, no. 3 (2006): 167–174. doi:10.1016/j.jphotobiol.2006.02.012.

Rauš, Karel, Stephan Pleschka, Peter Klein, Roland Schoop, and Peter Fisher. "Effect of an *Echinacea*-based hot drink versus oseltamivir in influenza treatment: A randomized, double-blind, double-dummy, multicenter, noninferiority clinical trial." *Current Therapeutic Research* 77 (2015): 66–72. doi:10.1016/j.curtheres.2015.04.001.

Safarabadi, Mehdi, Ehsanollah Ghaznavi-Rad, Abdolghader Pakniyat, Korosh Rezaie, and Ali Jadidi. "Comparing the effect of echinacea and chlorhexidine mouthwash on the microbial flora of intubated patients admitted to the intensive care unit." *Iranian Journal of Nursing and Midwifery Research* 22, no. 6 (2017): 481. doi:10.4103/ijnmr.ijnmr_92_16.

Samout, Noura, Amani Ettaya, Hafsia Bouzenna, Sana Ncib, Abdelfattah Elfeki, and Najla Hfaiedh. "Beneficial effects of *Plantago albicans* on high-fat diet-induced obesity in rats." *Biomedicine & Pharmacotherapy* 84 (2016): 1768–1775. doi:10.1016/j.biopha.2016.10.105.

Shikov, Alexander N., Olga N. Pozharitskaya, Valery G. Makarov, Dmitry V. Demchenko, and Evgenia V. Shikh. "Effect of *Leonurus cardiaca* oil extract in patients with arterial hypertension accompanied by anxiety and sleep disorders." *Phytotherapy Research* 25, no. 4 (2011): 540–543. doi:10.1002/ptr.3292.

Sienkiewicz, Monika, Monika Łysakowska, Edward Kowalczyk, Grażyna Szymańska, Ewa Kochan, Jolanta Krukowska, Jurek Olszewski, and Hanna Zielińska-Bliźniewska. "The ability of selected plant essential oils to enhance the action of recommended antibiotics against pathogenic wound bacteria." *Burns* 43, no. 2 (2017): 310–317. doi:10.1016/j.burns.2016.08.032.

Uzair, Bushra, Naheed Niaz, Asma Bano, Barkat Ali Khan, Naheed Zafar, Muhammad Iqbal, Riffat Tahira, and Fehmida Fasim. "Essential oils showing in vitro anti MRSA and synergistic activity with penicillin group of antibiotics." *Pakistan Journal of Pharmaceutical Sciences* 30 (2017). https://www.researchgate.net/publication/320299601_Essential_oils_showing_in_vitro_anti_MRSA_and_synergistic_activity_with_penicillin_group_of_antibiotics.

Vance, Katie M., David M. Ribnicky, Gerlinda E. Hermann, and Richard C. Rogers. "St. John's wort enhances the synaptic activity of the nucleus of the solitary tract." *Nutrition* 30, no. 7–8 (2014): S37–S42. doi:10.1016/j.nut.2014.02.008.

Verma, Rameshwar, Tushar Gangrade, Rakesh Punasiya, and Chetan Ghulaxe. "*Rubus fruticosus* (blackberry) use as an herbal medicine." *Pharmacognosy Reviews* 8, no. 16 (2014): 101. doi:10.4103/0973-7847.134239.

Wang, Jie, Xingjiang Xiong, and Bo Feng. "Effect of crataegus usage in cardiovascular disease prevention: An evidence-based approach." *Evidence-Based Complementary and Alternative Medicine* 2013 (2013). doi:10.1155/2013/149363.

Wu, Xiuxia, Xian Li, Zhongqin Dang, and Yunfei Jia. "Berberine demonstrates anti-inflammatory properties in *Helicobacter pylori*–infected mice with chronic gastritis by attenuating the Th17 response triggered by the B cell-activating factor." *Journal of Cellular Biochemistry* 119, no. 7 (2018): 5373–5381. doi:10.1002/jcb.26681.

Yang, Qiming, Meng Qi, Renchao Tong, Dandan Wang, Lili Ding, Zeyun Li, Cheng Huang, Zhengtao Wang, and Li Yang. "*Plantago asiatica* L. seed extract improves lipid accumulation and hyperglycemia in high-fat diet-induced obese mice." *International Journal of Molecular Sciences* 18, no. 7 (2017): 1393. doi:10.3390/ijms18071393.

Yin, Jun, Huili Xing, and Jianping Ye. "Efficacy of berberine in patients with type 2 diabetes mellitus." *Metabolism* 57, no. 5 (2008): 712–717. doi:10.1016/j.metabol.2008.01.013.

Yu, Hyeon-Hee, Kang-Ju Kim, Jeong-Dan Cha, Hae-Kyoung Kim, Young-Eun Lee, Na-Young Choi, and Yong-Ouk You. "Antimicrobial activity of berberine alone and in combination with ampicillin or oxacillin against methicillin-resistant *Staphylococcus aureus*." *Journal of Medicinal Food* 8, no. 4 (2005): 454–461. doi:doi.org/10.1089/jmf.2005.8.454.

Zakay-Rones, Zichria, Noemi Varsano, Moshe Zlotnik, Orly Manor, Liora Regev, Miriam Schlesinger, and Madeleine Mumcuoglu. "Inhibition of several strains of influenza virus in vitro and reduction of symptoms by an elderberry extract (*Sambucus nigra* L.) during an outbreak of influenza B Panama." *Journal of Alternative and Complementary Medicine* 1, no. 4 (1995): 361–369. doi:10.1089/acm.1995.1.361.

BOOKS

Breverton, Terry, Nicholas & Culpeper. *Breverton's Complete Herbal: A Book of Remarkable Plants and Their Uses.* London: Quercus, 2011.

Elpel, Thomas J. *Botany in a Day: The Patterns Method of Plant Identification: An Herbal Field Guide to Plant Families of North America.* Pony, MT: HOPS Press, 2018.

Falconi, Dina, and Wendy Hollender. *Foraging & Feasting: A Field Guide and Wild Food Cookbook.* Accord, NY: Botanical Arts Press, 2013.

Hoffmann, David. *Medical Herbalism: The Science and Practice of Herbal Medicine.* Accord, NY: Simon and Schuster, 2003.

Wood, Matthew David and Ryan. *The Earthwise Herbal Repertory: The Definitive Practitioner's Guide.* Berkeley, CA: North Atlantic Books, 2016.

ACKNOWLEDGMENTS

First I would like to thank Page Street Publishing, and especially my editor Sarah Monroe and copyeditor Jenna Nelson Patton, as well as the entire Page Street team, for helping me to bring my dream of publishing a book about medicinal herbs to reality. I am in awe that I have had such a tremendous opportunity. Sarah, thank you for holding my hand throughout the process!

To the herbalists who have made working in this field possible, I am forever in your debt. You have found a way to keep plant medicine alive in an increasingly industrialized world. To all the many herbalists, from well-known authors to folk and community herbalists—thank you, thank you, thank you. We are keeping plant medicine alive and well. This is good work.

To my nittygrittylife.com followers, if it weren't for your loyalty, encouraging words, thoughtful insights and inspiring questions this book wouldn't exist. You guys keep me learning every day!

To Mountain Rose Herbs, the great things that you do for the herbal community—and this herbalist in particular—should not go unmentioned. It is endlessly reassuring to know that there is a resource for beautiful herbs that I cannot grow or wildcraft myself.

To my friends and colleagues: I am blessed to move in the same circles as some amazing bloggers, authors and artists too numerous to mention, but I will give it a shot: Colleen C., Jess L., Kris B., Ann S., the triple Amys, Chris D., Susan V., Kathie L., Tessa Z., Quinn V., Dawn G., Megan C., Jan B., Tanya A., Janet G., Amanda I., Meredith F., Connie M., Shelle W., Angi S., Rachel A., Teri P. and Isis L. You ladies are so unbelievably awesome and keep this lady a little bit saner. To the Gather gals, your work perpetually inspires. To the Wondersmith—art and herbs, what more could I ask for in a friend. To my Wild Foodies peeps—foragers unite! To the amazing ladies that contributed photos, thank you for being an extra lens capturing the beautiful plants in this book. To all my friends elsewhere, you guys make this introvert come out of her shell—and I thank you for that!

To my kids, thanks for putting up with the "weird" mom. The mom that suddenly pulls over to take a closer look at some roadside plant, the mom that makes you drink fire cider and gargle sage and wouldn't be caught dead with a bottle of DayQuil. I do this all for you, and I love you dearly. Your wellness is my greatest focus.

To my extended family, thank you for supporting my ambitions and believing in me. I could not have done this without your love and cheerleading! I really have the best parents, sisters, grandparents, aunts, uncles, cousins and in-laws a girl could ask for.

To my husband, Stephen . . . I cannot adequately express in words how your support has allowed me to grow into being me. Your love for and belief in me feeds my soul. Also, thanks for letting me know before you mow the lawn so that I can collect my "weeds."

And to the plants . . . You are what this is all about. Thank you for the healing that you bring to the world.

ABOUT THE AUTHOR

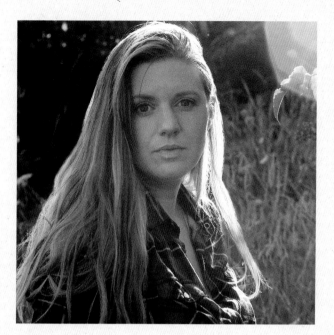

DEVON YOUNG lives with her husband and household of children on 20 acres on the westernmost edge of the Willamette Valley in Oregon. There they homestead, continually renovate a 100-year-old farmhouse and enjoy life on the peaceful banks of their favorite creek. A plant nerd from an early age, Devon finally pursued a formal education in complementary and alternative medicine at the American College of Healthcare Sciences, completing her degree in 2017. Her blog, nittygrittylife.com, is a resource for holistic, sustainable living with a focus on herbal medicine, foraging and the various aspects of homesteading, such as gardening, cooking from scratch and food preservation. Her work can also be seen at learningherbs.com, attainablesustainable.com, growforagecookferment.com, as well as the *Backwoods Home* magazine. Devon has an insatiable thirst for herbal knowledge and frequently can be located behind a mountain of books. If not creating, making, feeding, canning, cooking, seeing clients, writing, gardening or poking things with sticks, Devon can probably be found watching the reruns of the *Great British Baking Show* with her youngest daughter, trying to explain that *pâte à choux* has nothing to do with shoes.

INDEX